SHELTERING ARMS HOSPITAL:

A Centennial History (1889-1989), with Updates through 2006

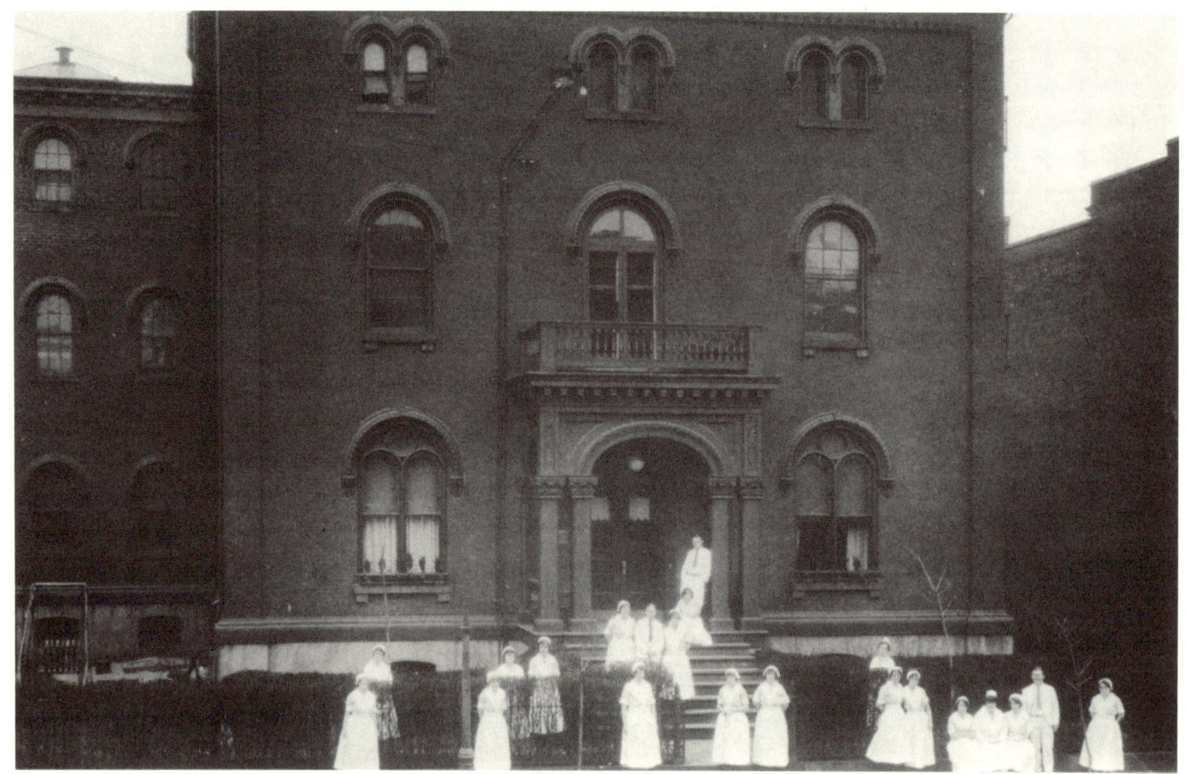

Sheltering Arms Hospital on Clay Street (1926).

A Centennial History (1889-1989)

SHELTERING ARMS HOSPITAL

with Updates through 2006

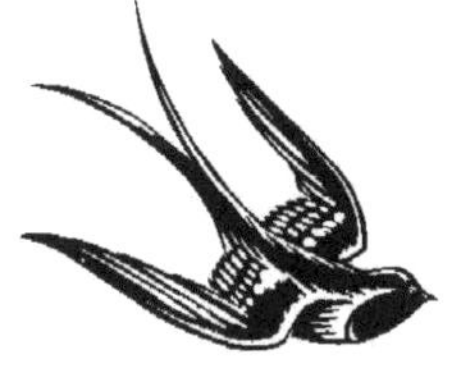

Anne Rutherford Lower

Printed in the United States of America by

THE AMERICAN BOOK COMPANY

Midlothian, Virginia

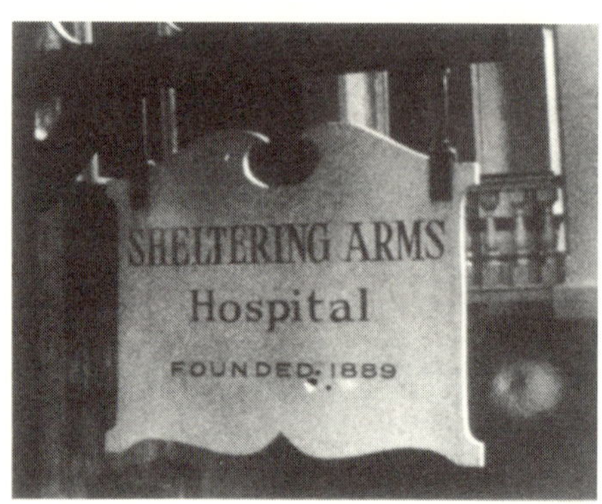

8254 Atlee Road, Mechanicsville, Virginia 23116

ISBN 0-9623370-0-5 (paper)
ISBN 0-9623370-1-3 (cloth)
Library of Congress Number 90-060051

Lower, Anne Rutherford
Sheltering Arms Hospital:
A Centennial History (1889-1998), with Updates through 2006

Printed in the United States of America by
The American Book Company
11020 Lady Allison La., Midlothian, VA 23113
804-241-1927 / Firstword1@aol.com

Third Printing, May, 2006

FOREWORD

On the celebration of the 100th anniversary of Sheltering Arms Hospital, this history, compiled by Anne Lower (Mrs. Richard R. Lower), presents an accurate record of this hospital's contributions to health care in Richmond during the past century.

Since its beginnings Sheltering Arms has admitted the less fortunate, the ill, and the maimed, regardless of their ability to pay. In a short space of time there developed an indescribable spirit in an environment where service was a privilege.

Since its inception, Sheltering Arms has been a community resource in which many citizens have had a part: the unselfish physicians, attending patients without remuneration; the dedicated nurses and staff, serving without counting the hours; the citizens and organizations continuing to give generous support; and, last but not least, the volunteers, young and old, who have considered it a privilege to give their time and talents in so many capacities through the years.

The best physicians in the city practiced at Sheltering Arms, and this great hospital acted as a meeting place for them. Most of the staff cared for their patients at the hospital with which they were affiliated; when at Sheltering Arms they would discuss medical and other problems; and a sense of camaraderie developed in that special setting.

As the demand for in-patient care for the indigent decreased, the hospital closed its acute care service. Much study and deliberation had led to the decision to become a comprehensive rehabilitation hospital. Like a stalwart patient, it has adapted well to the change, and its success has been phenomenal: today, it is one of the most outstanding rehabilitation facilities in the South.

As with people, institutions have a certain uniqueness and personality, and Anne Lower has found them at Sheltering

Arms. She has blended these with history, tradition and factual data, which together give the reader the real story of the hospital since its inception.

Even though Mrs. Lower has been a Richmonder only since 1965, she has participated in all facets of the hospital. She has served as president of the board, on virtually all of its committees, and is in constant contact with the inner workings of the hospital. Further, and probably more important, she was a vital force in convincing the board to convert the hospital to a comprehensive rehabilitation center. She is a tireless worker and a superb leader. Through months of meticulous research and communication with many who have been associated with the hospital throughout the years, she has given us a concise, readable and factual picture of the "hospital with a heart."

To her it was a work of love and to us it is a monument to a cherished institution.

Charles M. Caravati, M.D.
Former member, Board of Directors
July 1989

CONTENTS

The Mission of Sheltering Arms

A non-profit institution operating with public support since 1889, Sheltering Arms' mission is to provide needed health care and enhance the quality of life of persons experiencing disabilities.

Sheltering Arms seeks to fulfill its mission by:

- Providing comprehensive physical rehabilitation in a continuum of services which enable the individual to achieve optimal potential;
- Providing care to persons who can benefit from the services regardless of their ability to pay;
- Continuing a tradition of concern for the dignity and human needs of the individual;
- Assuring quality care in a cost effective manner;
- Providing an environment in which personnel are enabled to attain high standards of accomplishment and personal fulfillment;
- Developing educational and research programs to advance the knowledge and science of physical medicine and rehabilitation;
- Promoting public awareness of its services and positive attitudes concerning the needs and capacities of persons with disabilities.

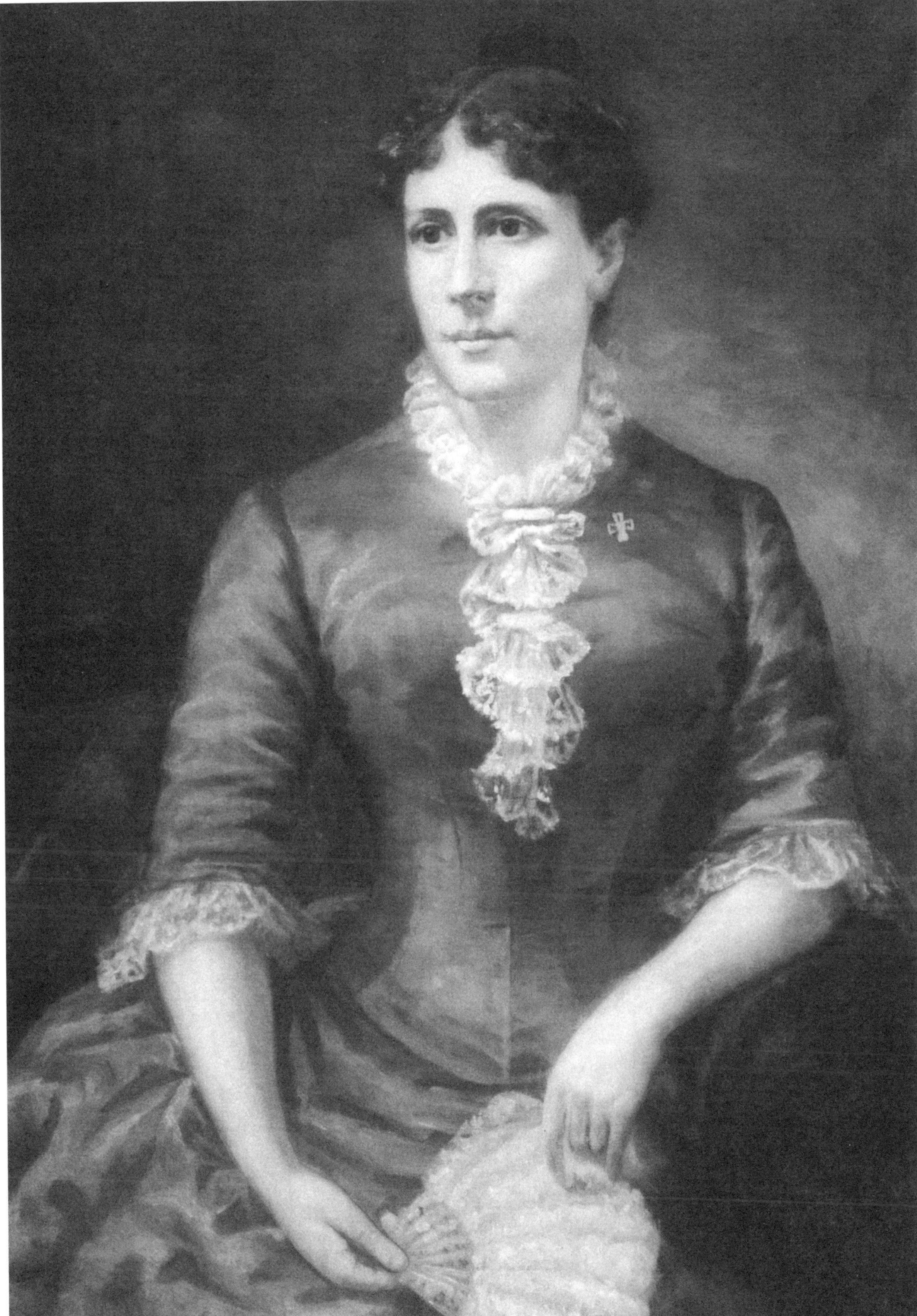

Dedicated to
Florence Robertson Givens
teacher, musician, gardener
who brought joy to life
and gave us courage.

PREFACE

AS SOMEONE NEW TO RICHMOND in 1965, I first heard of Sheltering Arms when my young children asked to take canned goods to school as Thanksgiving donations for the Hospital. My formal introduction came a few years later when I became a member of the Board of Managers. I have since watched Sheltering Arms develop and respond to the necessity of change. And I could not fail to note a magical quality about the Hospital. This is what I wish to place in the perspective of time, now, as Sheltering Arms celebrates its centennial year.

In reconstructing the story, I have sought to sense what the world was like to people of long ago. The Sheltering Arms personalities of bygone years were stars around which formed constellations. Where did their energy come from? And how has it been passed on to succeeding generations? There was definitely a contagious spirit about service to Sheltering Arms. Morton G. Thalhimer, Sr., a devoted board member and president, identified it as a "disease," which, once caught, could never be cured.

The spirit of Sheltering Arms began, of course, with its founder, Rebekah Peterkin. It was amplified by other dynamic personalities through the years, passing from generation to generation, and it pervades our very beings today. The dream that came to one woman a century ago is now manifested in hundreds of people. Why? Because the mission of Rebekah Peterkin and Sheltering Arms has remained true: to help others in time of need regardless of their ability to pay.

Three things are especially significant to me in the hundred-year life of Sheltering Arms: the dignity of the individual, the role of women, and the value of volunteerism.

It seems to me that a great rise in industrialization and a shrinking of the place of the individual human being occurred toward the end of the nineteenth century. As our nation surged forward industrially, the "little guy" was in jeopardy. Certainly, as Rebekah Peterkin observed in Richmond, he was precariously positioned in terms of receiving good health care. Now, at the close of the twentieth century, we are anxious that the age of technology may again diminish the individual. As a noble institution, Sheltering Arms has sought to care for the individual and respect his or her dignity; this has been and continues to be its hallmark.

In the South in the 1880s and 1890s, many women were beginning to break out of traditional molds and establish their own identities. Not every woman married and raised a family. What, then, was actually available for women to do? The great professions of teaching and nursing appealed to the feminine instincts of nurturing and caring. Perhaps, for independent, often unmarried women, nursing and teaching were the primary callings. At Sheltering Arms the nurses have always been exemplary of their profession and held in high esteem, the epitome of excellent care, lovingly administered.

Another social fact of life toward the end of the last century was that women, including those who did have a husband and children, were searching for ways to use their energy to relieve human suffering. Women were choosing to do volunteer work in areas of perceived need: for orphans, the mentally ill, the poor, and the sick. Volunteerism appealed to people of all walks of life, and this American phenomenon was never more fully displayed than at Sheltering Arms Hospital.

Volunteers have been essential in the Hospital and in raising money in the community. Sheltering Arms has inspired both men and women to seek donations for patient care, and millions of dollars in private funds have been contributed for the public good. Volunteerism is often a response to gratitude for one's blessings, and Sheltering Arms encourages voluntary participation and enjoyment in the act of doing something for someone else.

In our city of monuments, we build monuments in our hearts to the spiritual leaders of Sheltering Arms, both past and present, and the constellations of committed souls who surround them.

A.R.L.

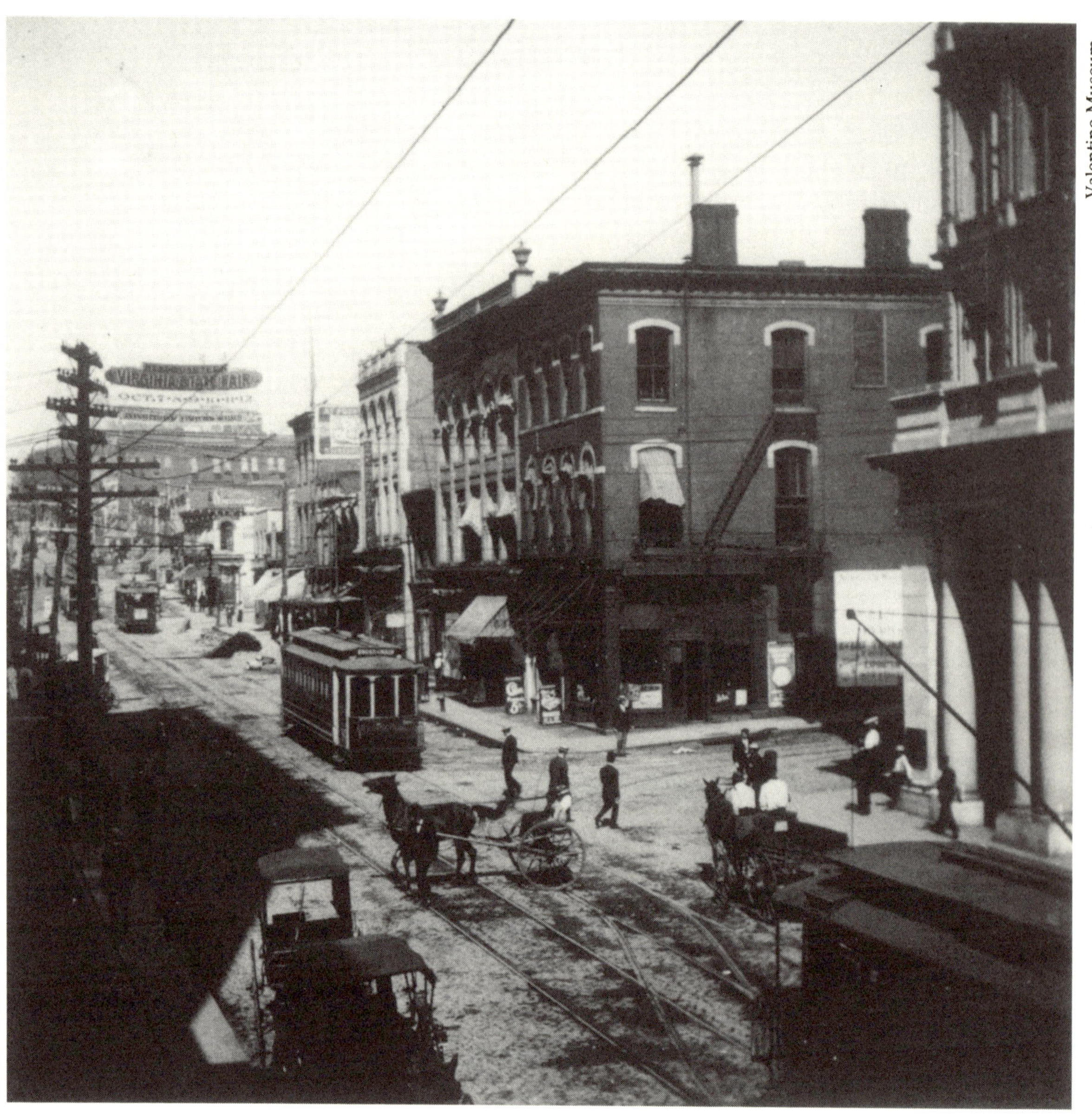

Valentine Museum

Main Street in Richmond, Virginia, about 1890.

1

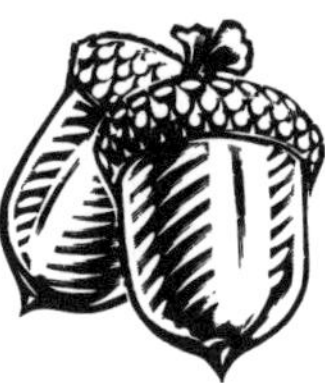

The Beginnings (1889-1894)

THE STORY OF SHELTERING ARMS HOSPITAL is a story of caring. It begins in Richmond, Virginia, in the late 1880s, an era when the South was just beginning to awaken from the shock of Appomattox. Industry was in a period of expansion. By 1887, many small, family-run firms—such as C.F. Sauer, Miller and Rhoads, Crawford Manufacturing, and Albemarle Paper—were just being established.

During this era of growth, the need for health care was magnified by the rapidly increasing population, from 51,038 in 1870 to 81,388 in 1890. With it came an explosion of industrial injuries. Newspaper accounts of the day have preserved for us the anguish and pain of life in an emerging urban area: children injured by runaway horses and buggies, hands wrenched in machinery, gruesome railroad accidents, and the pain and terror of fire.

As Dr. Charles Caravati notes in his *Medicine in Richmond, 1900 to 1975*, even in the more prosperous neighborhoods, living and sanitary conditions in the late 19th century were quite primitive. The water supply, from the James River, was untreated. Hundreds of workers were employed by the many southern railroads, two of which, the C. & O. and R.F. & P., had large shops in Richmond. The "electric car," which began operating on an experimental twelve-mile track in Richmond in 1887, caused confusion and mayhem on the city streets.

It was in this period of bustling transition and increasing need that a young woman, Rebekah Peterkin, decided to turn her observant concern into actual care for those who needed it most. As the daughter of Joshua Peterkin, D.D., rector of St.

James's Episcopal Church at Fifth and Marshall Streets, Rebekah knew the suffering of those around her. Her vision was to help the weakest of them—the poor, injured or sick—regain their health, their jobs, and their self-respect.

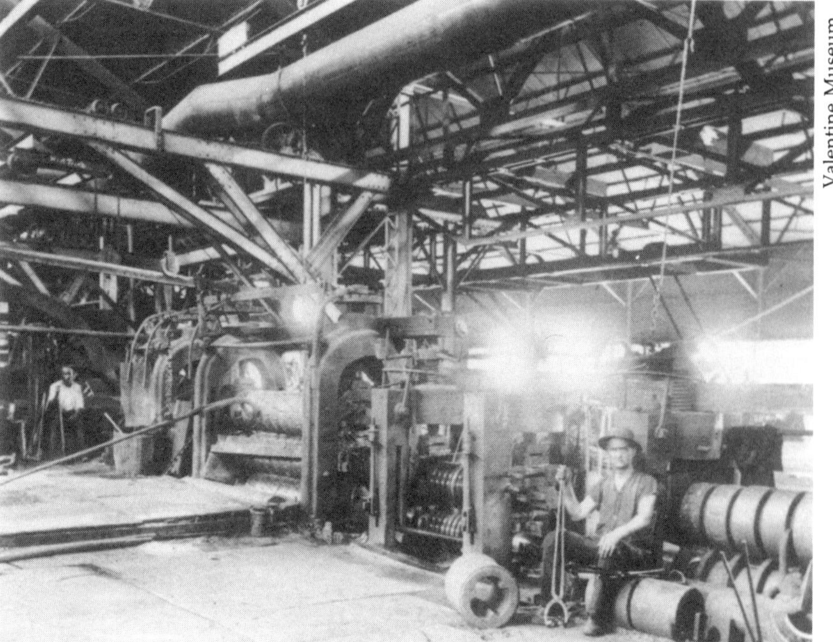

Valentine Museum

Industry was expanding in the 1890s and the Tredegar Iron Works was a large employer.

Far away, in New York City, the Order of The King's Daughters had just been formed by Margaret Bottome with the help of her friends, wealthy women who shared the desire to help others less fortunate than themselves. In 1886 this group of ten women had organized a sisterhood of service to others based upon the Biblical text (Mark 10:45) "not to be ministered unto, but to minister." Their motto is still recited at meetings:

Look up and not down,
Look forward and not back,
Look out and not in,
And lend a hand.

At first they were called "The Ten," but that appellation was soon changed to "circle," and the new circles were not limited to ten members. That kernel of faith and the willingness to volunteer radiated far beyond New York City. By 1887 the inspiration had spread to Richmond. The purpose of The King's Daughters had strong appeal and practical application for Rebekah Peterkin and she was swift to urge her church sewing circle to become the first Richmond chapter of King's Daughters, the third in Virginia. While three other small hospitals served the city at this time—Retreat for the Sick, St. Luke's, and Old Dominion Hospital—Sheltering Arms would offer free care for the white working poor.

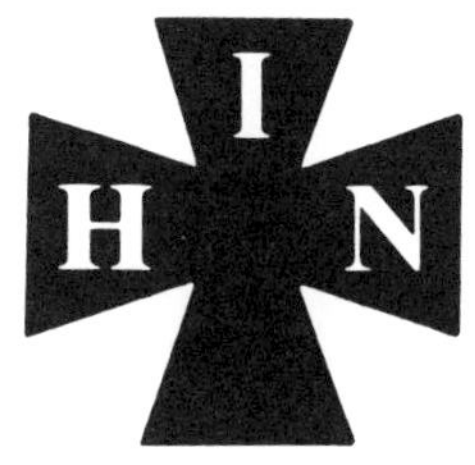

The symbol and pin of the International Order of King's Daughters and Sons.

With her sewing circle and a few friends, particularly among the physicians of that day, Rebekah Peterkin forged her conviction and her compassion into the dream of a free hospital. Money was scarce during the 1890s, and many charitable institutions were founded in Richmond during this period. Undaunted courage and great faith were the sole capital of Miss Peterkin's enterprise at first. She must have been an inspiring leader, for she so infused enthusiasm into her young friends that even her death two years later did not deter their efforts.

The St. James's sewing circle was called the Central Circle. The original ten members included Mrs. William Cole, Miss Nannie Davies, Miss Mary Greenhow, Mrs. Mary May, Mrs. Robert Rennolds, Miss Annie Sheppard, Mrs. John G. Wayt, and the sisters Miss Hettie Taylor and Mrs. Walter Williams. Rebekah Peterkin was their leader.

Below: Alice Taylor Williams, one of the original ten women in the Central Circle of King's Daughters, shown here with her husband Walter Williams, and children Carrington, Isabel, and Walter, Jr., in 1890s.

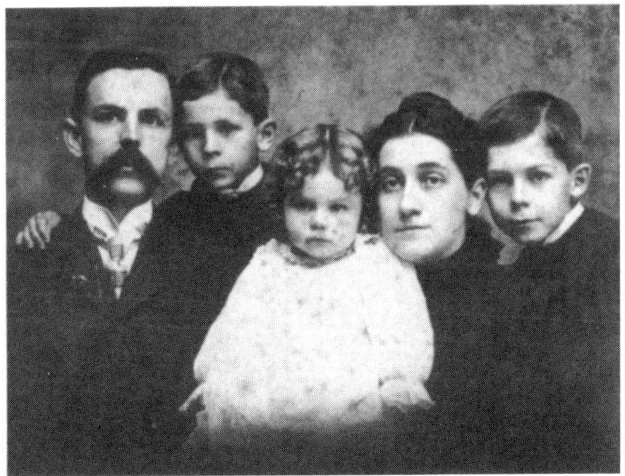

At thirty-eight years of age in 1887, Rebekah was considered a woman of rare personal charm and intelligence. She was determined to establish a hospital to care for the "respectable poor" in the area of downtown Richmond. Her patients would be men and women who could not work for reasons of ill health, yet neither could they afford medical care. "Sheltering Arms" was a perfect name for the service Rebekah envisioned. It is no coincidence that it was the same name as the hospital for sick miners and railroad workers which her brother, Bishop George William Peterkin, had founded in Hansford, West Virginia, the year before.

With little except the Central Circle's willingness to get the idea started, Miss Peterkin approached Dr. Edwin Gilliam Booth of Carter's Grove. Dr. Booth owned The Clifton House, an old boarding house at 107 North Fourteenth Street, between Ross and Franklin Streets, that had become a Home for the Friendless under the guidance of Mrs. Lucy A. Booth. The house, built around 1778, was once fashionable and elegant, but was now in need of cleaning and repair. Miss Peterkin received permission

Dr. Edwin Booth generously donated the Clifton House, first home of Sheltering Arms Hospital. It was located east of the Governor's Mansion on Fourteenth Street.

Right: Bettie Ellett, confined to a wheelchair, found a home in Sheltering Arms from 1889 to 1918.

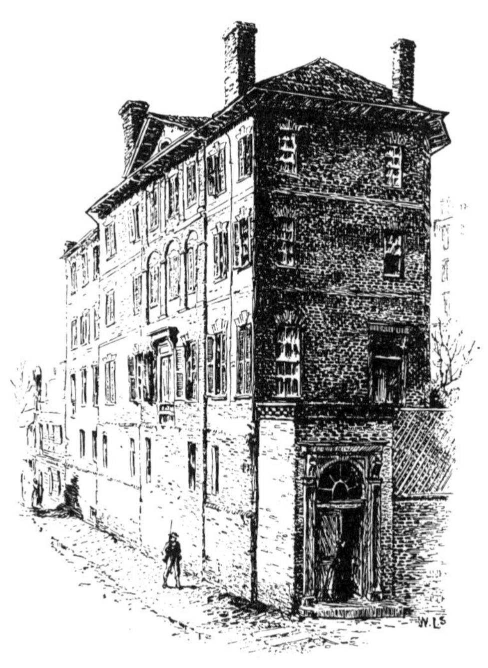

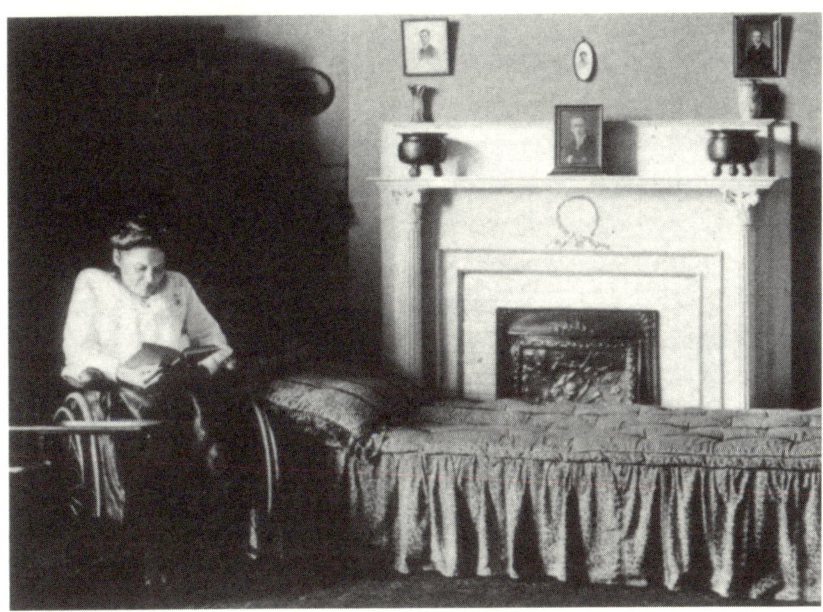

to use the Clifton House free of charge for one year, and for the sum of $5 a month thereafter.

The young women of Central Circle quickly set to work to realize their dream. They begged funds and supplies from friends, and made the first blankets by sewing newspapers between yellow cotton covers. The tradition of frugality at Sheltering Arms had its genesis then and there. The women also collected broken and discarded kitchen utensils, seeking help from a sympathetic plumber who would solder them back together so that they could be used again. The women themselves mopped the floors and scrubbed the walls of the old house to make it ready for opening day—February 13, 1889.

The Hospital's first patient was a Mrs. Kellam, the widow of a Confederate veteran, who was transferred from the City Almshouse to the Hospital in a horse-drawn "black mariah." The Almshouse had furnished the only free medical care at this time in a city of about 80,000 inhabitants.

Rebekah herself brought in a little lame girl, Bettie Ellett, who became the beloved "daughter" of the Hospital, and remained living there until her death twenty-nine years later.

Dr. Moses Hoge, Jr., was persuaded to become the first doctor for Sheltering Arms. By volunteering his services, he established a tradition of physicians and surgeons who offered their care free of charge to the patients of Sheltering Arms.

Sheltering Arms enjoyed an affiliation with the schools of medicine. Here, the 1894 faculty of the University College of Medicine, including Hunter H. McGuire, front row center; Jacob Michaux, directly behind; and Moses D. Hoge, Jr., behind and to Dr. Michaux's right.

Among other leading doctors who gave their support to the fledgling hospital were James B. McCaw, Hunter H. McGuire, Lewis C. Bosher, C. V. Carrington, Stuart McGuire, W. T. Oppenhimer, J. H. White, and George Ross. These and many other Richmonders were influential in getting the Hospital started, and a charter of incorporation was granted on March 2, 1891.

An executive board of ladies who devoted heart and purse to Sheltering Arms included Mrs. J. H. Claiborne, president; Miss Frances Branch Scott, first vice president; Mrs. W. T. Pemberton, second vice president; Mrs. L. B. Janney, third vice president; Mrs. George T. King, treasurer; Miss Annie Sheppard, secretary; Miss Annie W. Moore, recording secretary; Miss Anna Boykin, Mrs. Edmund D. T. Myers, and Mrs. A. L. Wellford, members at large.

This group, also referred to as the "executive committee," met weekly at Sheltering Arms and was responsible for the management of the Hospital. Funds were always scarce and announcements were made regularly to the committee requesting items needed for medical care, as well as for the everyday needs of patients and staff. Donations were carefully recorded in the minutes and reflect the scope of the members' efforts: a set of chamber furniture, fireplace fenders, mattress, clothes, firewood, a bottle of whiskey, a barrel of flour, blankets, and an invalid's chair (gift of Dr. Hoge). Mrs. King reported she had purchased twenty-seven loads of coal from the C. & O. Railroad, and a Mr. Hawes donated the hauling of the coal.

In the first year of operating Sheltering Arms in the Clifton House, the patient cost per day had been about sixty-seven cents. The Hospital's managers spent $1245 of an income of $1417 to care for fewer than sixty patients, whose average stay was thirty days. It is reported that an anonymous check for $5000 literally sent the executive committee into hysterics.

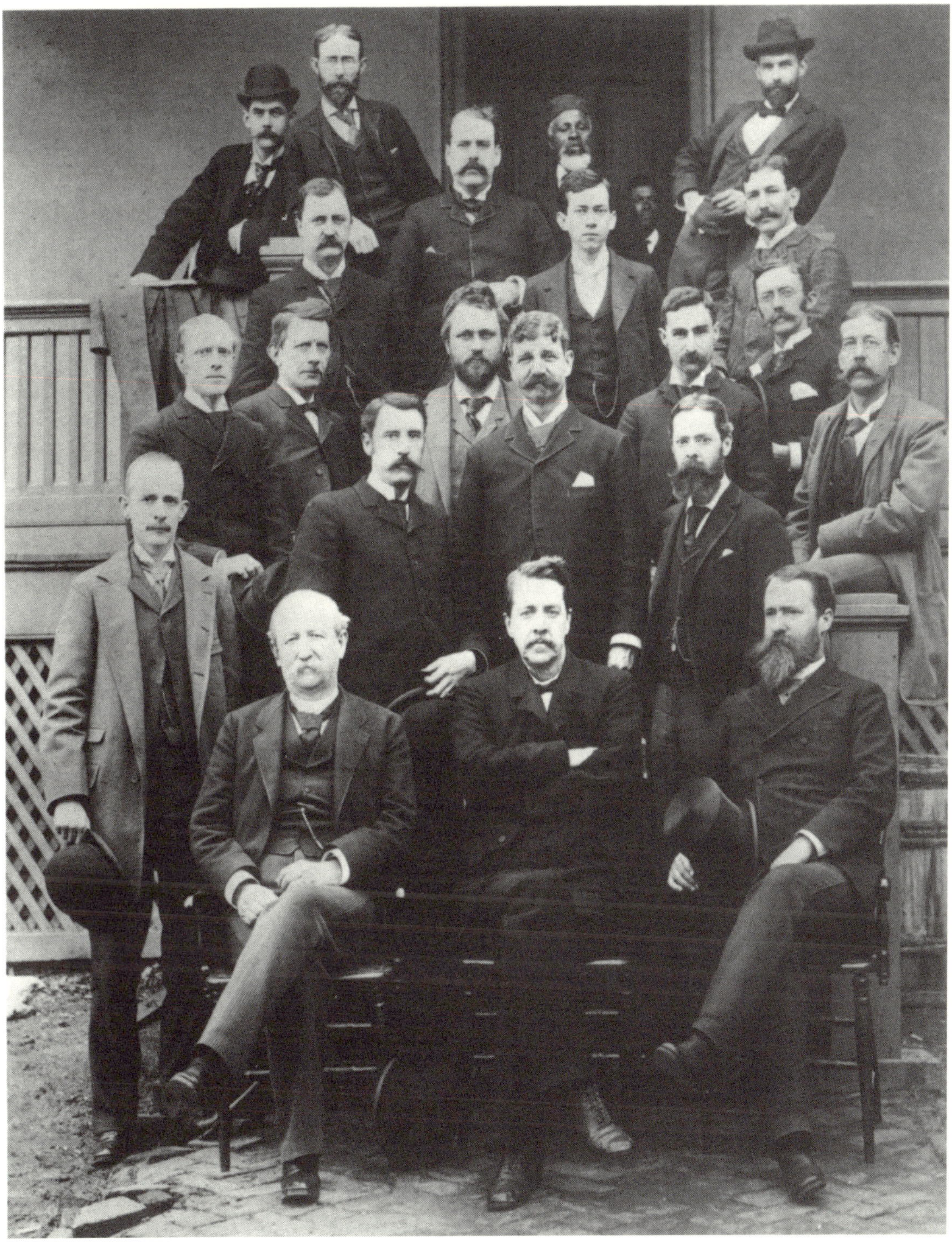

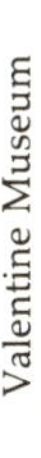
Valentine Museum

Capitalizing on the space not needed for patients in the Clifton House, The King's Daughters set up a lunchroom on the first floor, the profit from which was used to run the Hospital.

The charter had also established a men's board of directors to oversee the financial affairs of the Hospital. The original board included C. V. Meredith, president; Dr. Moses D. Hoge, Jr.; George E. Crawford; John W. Fergusson; Reverend L. B. Turnbull; Henry S. Hutzler; J. A. Curry; D. O. Davis; L. B. Tatum; and William Ryan.

Rebekah Peterkin died in her forty-second year, 1891, when Sheltering Arms Hospital was little more than two years old. For a time, it seemed that Sheltering Arms might die with her. Then a good friend and another King's Daughter, Mrs. A. D. Landerkin, suggested the formation of a general board of all King's Daughters circle leaders. Perhaps the first problem facing the ladies was a tenable building to replace the decrepit Clifton House. One writer reported that Dr. James McCaw offered his old house, but the plan was abandoned because the neighbors objected!

A mass meeting was held in the Academy of Music, at which Dr. Hunter H. McGuire suggested that the doctors pledge $100 each. With the aid of the board of directors, enough funds were raised for a down payment ($13,500) on the stately Georgian mansion at 1008 East Clay Street, built in 1854 by tobacco manufacturer William H. Grant.

A group of leading citizens saw the need for an endowment fund for the future, to which bequests from wills could be donated. Among those original donors were Abram Levy, E. A. Saunders, Moses Millhiser, and Dr. Moses Hoge. It was they who had raised the down payment for the Grant House.

But even with a new home to its name, Sheltering Arms did not move immediately. It remained on Fourteenth Street until September 1893, and then abruptly closed for more than a year. Perhaps the severe depression, the worst since 1837, was one reason for the delay. Another reason was that the board of Sheltering Arms needed time to consider an 1892 proposal of a group of physicians and surgeons to unite with them in estab-

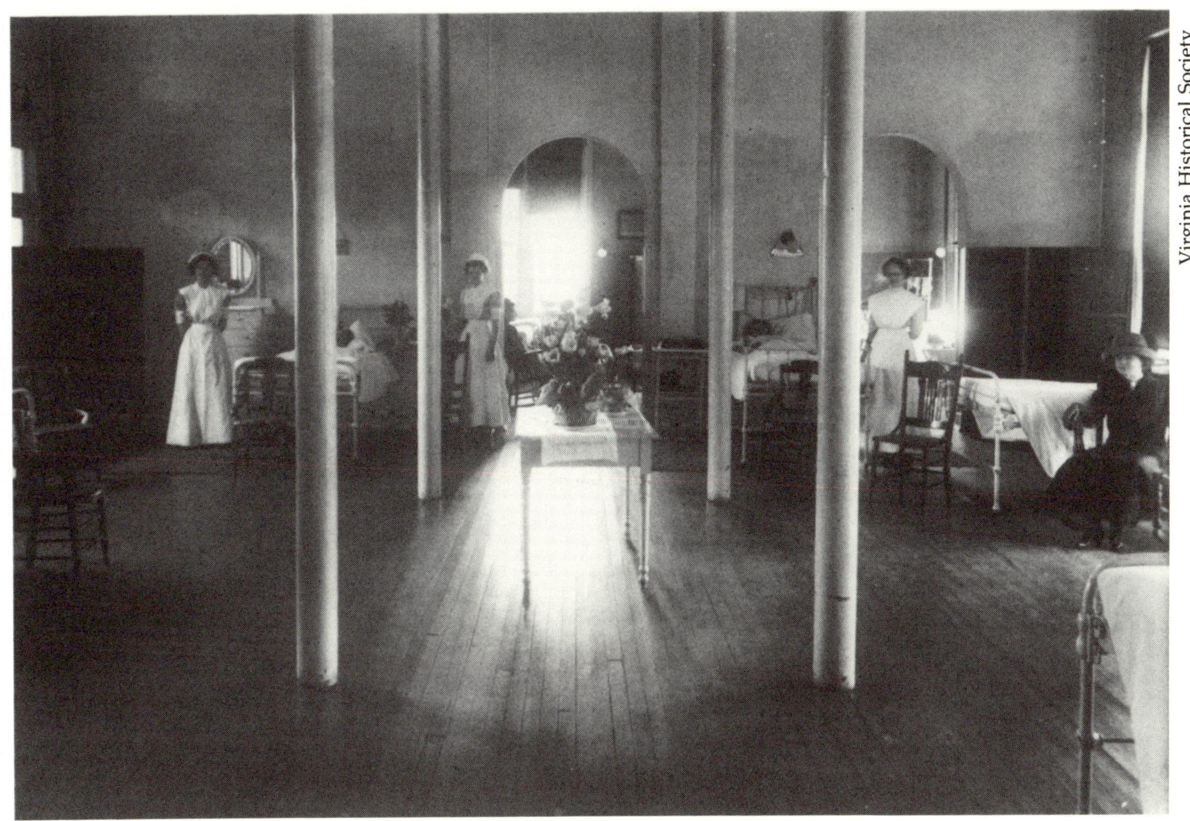

Virginia Historical Society

A ward of Sheltering Arms in the Grant House on Clay Street.

lishing the Virginia Hospital. The board eventually rejected the proposal in 1893.

Finally, Sheltering Arms Hospital was moved up the hill to Clay Street. The new location offered a beautiful view of the countryside beyond the Shockoe Valley to the northeast.

The King's Daughters themselves scoured and painted their new hospital until the rooms were "sweet and clean and ready for patients." The building was dedicated on November 20, 1894, with clergy of all denominations in attendance. The Right Reverend George William Peterkin, Rebekah's brother, delivered the invocation and was assisted in the dedication by the Reverend Moses D. Hoge, Rabbi Edward N. Calisch, and the Reverend George Cooper. The minutes of that event, now yellowed and crumbling, record in a spidery hand the offerings brought for this occasion by the "lady" board members: coffee, chocolate cakes, fancy breads, beaten biscuits, a cut of loaf sugar, and orange crackers.

Sheltering Arms was now firmly established in Richmond. From the dream of a young woman in the 1880s, with the faith and hard work of her friends, had arisen a great institution of caring.

2

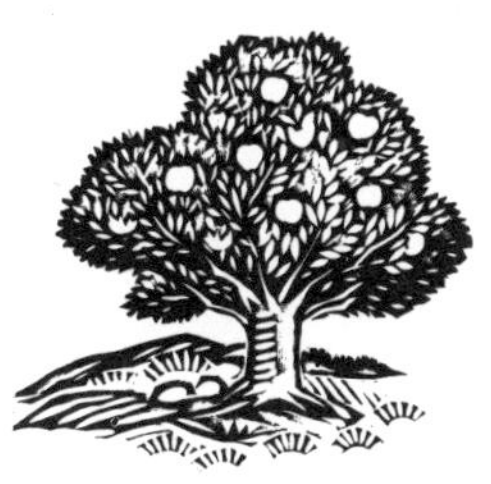

Foundations Grow, Roots Establish
(1895-1957)

AMONG THE FIRST OF MANY who devoted their lives to helping the needy at Sheltering Arms, Miss Frances Branch Scott served as first vice president of the executive board until 1911, then led the board as president for another twenty-seven years until her death on March 21, 1937. She, together with Mrs. George T. King, Mrs. Ramon Garcin, Miss Sally Archer Anderson, Mrs. William White, Mrs. W. P. Wood, and Mrs. S. Marshall Taylor, were members of the executive board in the early years of Sheltering Arms.

It was this board's duty to decide who would be admitted to the Hospital. At a meeting in January 1895, the Sick Committee of the board reported on its decisions, and in the spring of 1895 the first male patient was admitted. By summer a separate ward for male patients was opened on the third floor of the Grant building.

By 1895 the board had ratified a constitution and bylaws. The minutes of March 15, 1895, reflect the decision to have a young physician reside at Sheltering Arms as an "interne." There were thirteen patients in house on that date. By the next year, Dr. Hoge came before the board and asked that he "be allowed to select the interne, who comes this year from the class of '96 at the University College of Medicine" (merged with Medical College of Virginia in 1913). "As Dr. Hoge is a member of the Faculty of that College the ladies agreed that he should select the interne, provided he select a quiet and orderly young man, as well as one capable and proficient in his profession."

A "pupil" nurse program was begun in conjunction with Old Dominion Hospital whereby student nurses would rotate

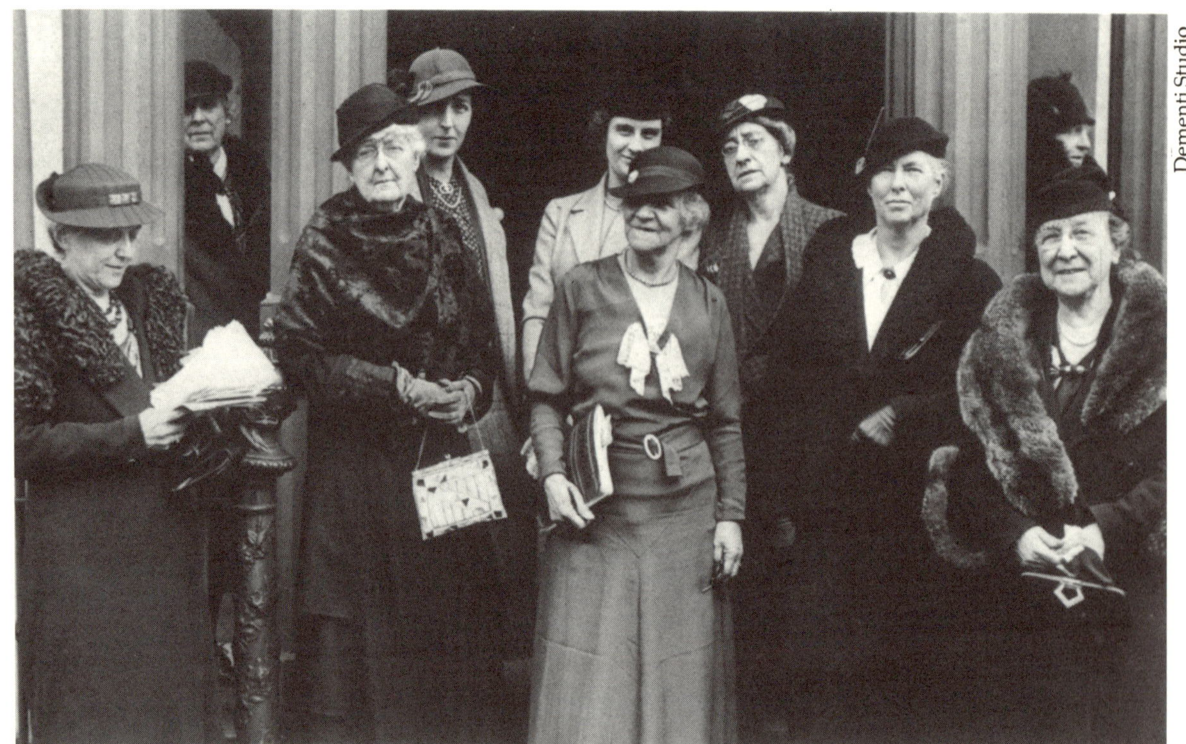

Dementi Studio

duty through Sheltering Arms every three months, receiving room, board, and laundry, with time set aside for leisure. In exchange, the sum of $6.00 a month would be paid to Old Dominion.

In 1894, when it was becoming difficult for Sheltering Arms to take patients considered incurable, board member Miss Mary Tinsley Greenhow felt so keen a sympathy for them that she was instrumental in establishing the Virginia Home for Incurables on Governor Street, later to become The Virginia Home, in Byrd Park. Miss Greenhow herself had been permanently crippled by a fall from a horse.

The minutes of December 20, 1895, recorded "The New Rules for Admission: a reliable person must state that the applicant is in needy circumstances and is not properly cared for at home; the applicant cannot have contagious or incurable diseases."

By 1896, the executive committee was seeking $500 from City Council for support of Sheltering Arms, as well as an appropriation from the State. In 1897 more than 100 patients received care at Sheltering Arms. In those years, too, it was the custom to close the Hospital for August and September, not only to give the staff a much needed vacation, but also to limit expenses when funds were running low.

The treasurer, Mrs. King, had worked miracles. By 1898, she was able to pay off two debts of one thousand dollars each, as well as the mortgage for the Clay Street building. Some months, however, the treasurer's report looked discouraging, since the Hospital needed both a new furnace and an elevator before winter. In her 75-year *History of Sheltering Arms*, Eda Carter Williams described this devoted exchequer of Sheltering Arms' funds as possessing the rare combination of a shrewd financier and the faith and zeal of a missionary.

The turn of the century found Rebekah Peterkin's mother at the helm of the Hospital, where she presided until her death in 1910. Since the death of both her daughter and her husband, she had maintained the family home on Leigh Street.

Far left: Executive Board of ladies who managed Sheltering Arms' day to day operation: front row, Mrs. Ramon Garcin, Miss Frances Branch Scott, Mrs. George T. King, Mrs. W. P. Wood, and Mrs. Pauline L. Thalhimer; back row, second from left, Mrs. Edward C. Anderson, Mrs. William Frazier, Mrs. S. Marshall Taylor.

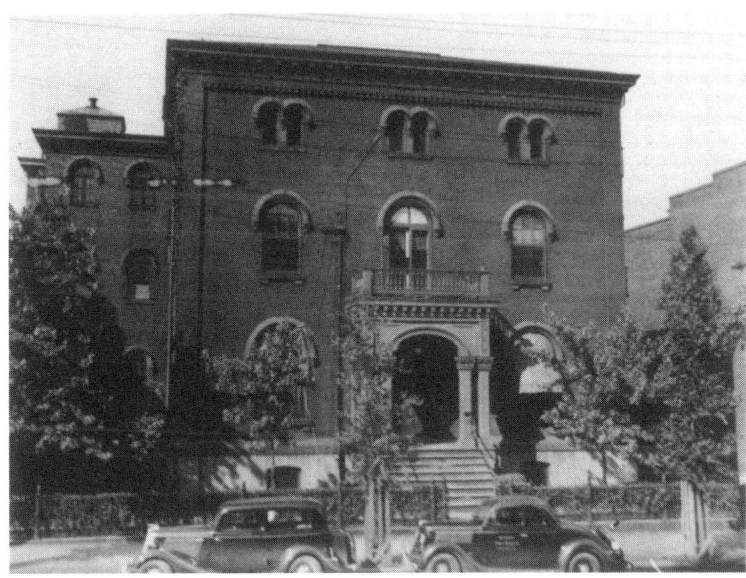

Near left: A haven of mercy from 1894 to 1965: Sheltering Arms in the stately Georgian mansion built by William H. Grant.

In 1904 the first session of Sheltering Arms' own nurses training school was held under the direction of Miss Mary Whitehead. The school was to graduate dedicated nurses who served with honor through the years in many hospitals, wearing their Sheltering Arms caps with pride. A number of them elected to remain at Sheltering Arms. The Hospital was always proud of its nurses, who exemplified the highest ideals of the nursing profession.

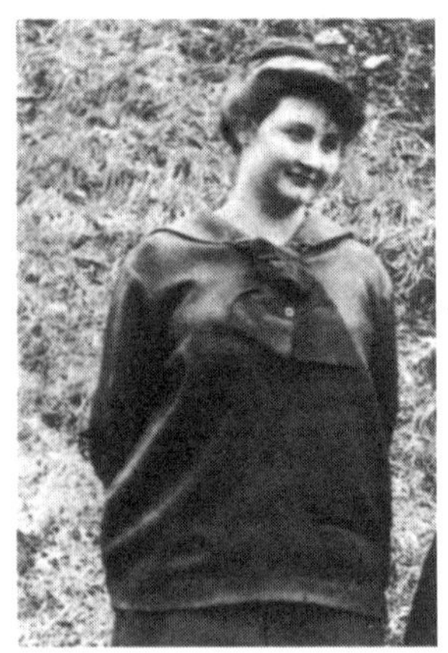

Clara Humphries as a young woman; she gave much of her life to The King's Daughters in West Virginia and Richmond.

Until they could obtain a residence of their own, these nurses lived on the third floor of the Hospital, described in the 1906 Yearbook as follows: ". . . passing through the portico, we enter a wide and lofty hall, running clear to double porches in the rear, from whence is a view, not only of grassy lawn, but miles of country outside the city limits, where fresh air has uninterrupted sweep. The rooms are large and airy, none containing more than four cots, for every effort is made to make the place homelike and cheery."

In addition to their board and lodging, students now received $15 a month. This allowance was not given as payment, but for uniforms, laundry, and textbooks. Please note the "hours of duty": students were on day duty from 7 a.m. to 7 p.m., with four hours off duty for rest and study. Five hours on Sunday. Students were on night duty for two months each year, and the hours were from 7 p.m. to 7 a.m., with two evenings off each month.

Lighter moments for the hard-working nursing students at Sheltering Arms, in the 1920s.

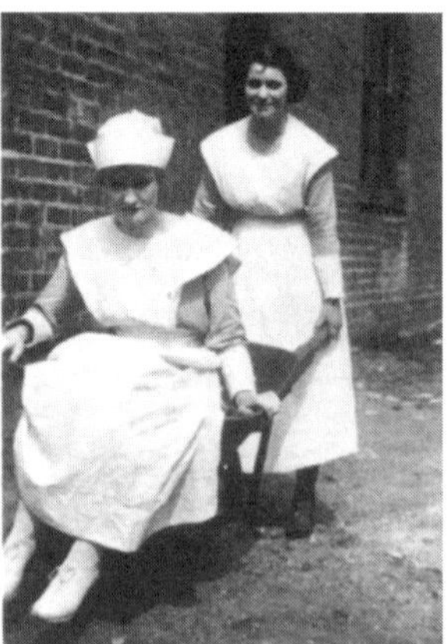

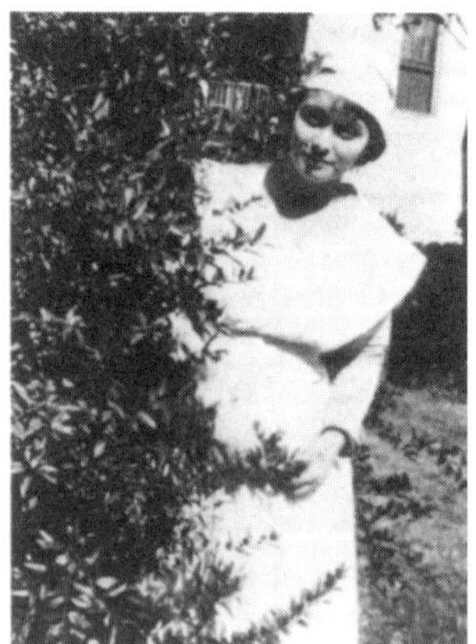

It was during this period that the Hospital's endowment fund began to attract attention as a worthy charitable cause. The 1906 Yearbook says "liberal" contributors were Edmund B. Addison, Mrs. Russell Robinson, and Mrs. John Addison. Many people remembered Sheltering Arms in their wills, among them a Captain Babcock, John Pope, Major Lewis Ginter, Mrs. T. C. Williams, E. A. Saunders, Moses Millhiser, Abram Levy, Robert S. Bosher, Mrs. S. R. Parker, T. W. Wood, and Emmanuel Millhiser of Richmond; Mrs. Elizabeth Waller of Williamsburg; and a Mr. Parish of Culpeper County.

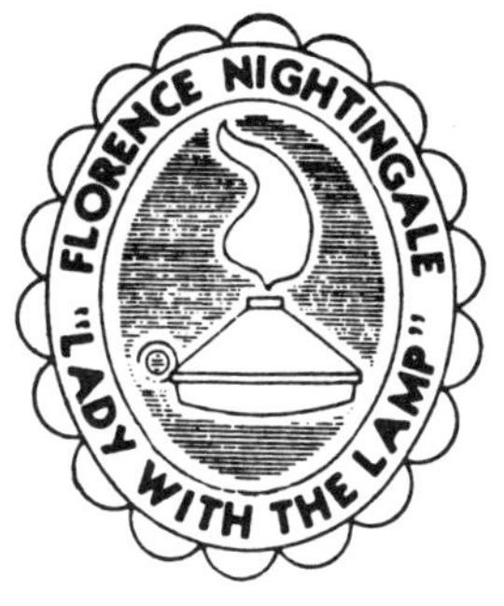

Logo of the Florence Nightingale Circle, the first Sheltering Arms auxiliary, established in 1910 to support the nursing staff.

Important events that occurred in this period of Sheltering Arms' history resulted in the establishment of other health care institutions. In 1908 it was discovered that a fifteen-year-old girl, a patient at Sheltering Arms, had tuberculosis. Since Sheltering Arms could not accept patients with contagious diseases, nor were there facilities for tubercular patients in any other hospital in Richmond, Miss Frances Branch Scott gathered her friends to discuss what could be done to help such patients. From their musings, Pine Camp Sanatorium and the Richmond Tuberculosis Association were born.

Also at Miss Scott's suggestion, Miss Josephine Sizer and Miss Sally Archer Anderson organized the Florence Nightingale auxiliary in 1910. Over the years, the Florence Nightingale Circle continued to help in the maintenance and renovation of both the Hospital and the nurses' quarters.

In 1911 Miss Scott succeeded Mrs. Peterkin as president of the executive board, sometimes called "the lady board of managers." It was Frances Branch Scott who guided the Hospital through the years of the First World War (1914-1918), when wards were crowded with members of soldiers' families. The number of newborn babies soon exceeded the supply of bassinets, and bureau drawers and soap boxes were used to bed them.

During the severe influenza epidemic that nearly decimated this country in 1918, Sheltering Arms Hospital was converted to the care of "flu" victims, as was the nearby John Marshall High School. Beds were placed in the offices and halls of

Sheltering Arms, and lay volunteers helped the staff cope with the tremendous overflow during this emergency.

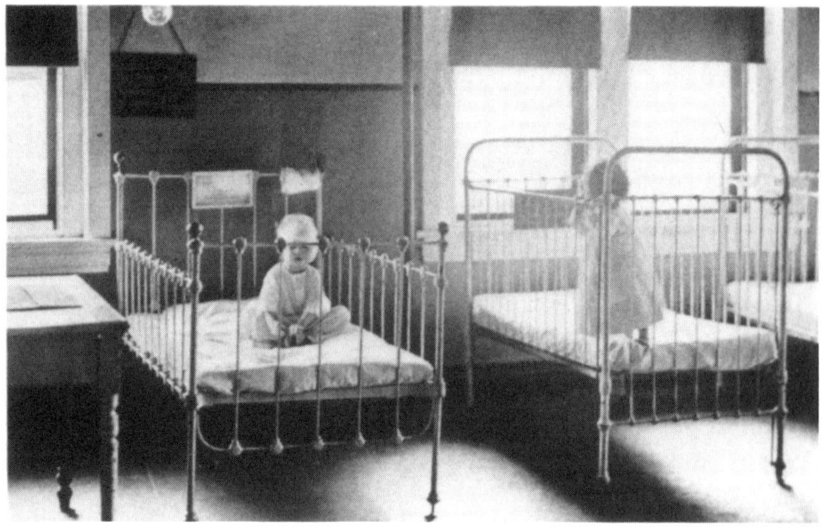

Upper: Children's ward at the Hospital.

Lower: 1925 invitation to Founders Day.

Right: Miss Frances Branch Scott was a long-time leader of Sheltering Arms, dedicated to the Hospital's work from 1891 to 1937.

Hospital records show that Sheltering Arms cared for 652 patients in 1917. By the next year, Sheltering Arms had grown to 52 beds. At this time The King's Daughters were operating a summer home in Charles City County, where convalescents could get an additional two weeks' rest after leaving the hospital. The Instructive Visiting Nurses Association was especially helpful with follow-up work so that a patient's hospital stay could be reduced.

Sheltering Arms Hospital
Richmond, Virginia

You are cordially invited to be present at the Thirty-Sixth Anniversary of the founding of the Sheltering Arms Hospital, Friday, February 13th, 1925, at noon. The usual exercises will be followed by a public reception at which light refreshments will be served.

Governor Trinkle will make the address.

No. Patients in 1924,	1,073	
No. Days Treatment,	17,097	Miss F. B Scott, President
Average No. Each Day,	50	Mrs. O. J. Sands, Rec. Sec'y
Cost Per Day Per Patient,	$1.92	Mrs. Levin Joynes, Cor. Sec'y
No. Births,	75	Mrs. Geo. T. King, Treasurer
No. Deaths,	24	Miss N. J. Curtis, Sup't
Entire Cost of Maintenance,	$31,102.51	Dr. Margaret Nolting, Med. Dir.
Value of Gifts of All Kinds,	$ 1,500.00	
Receipts from All Sources,	$32,210.31	

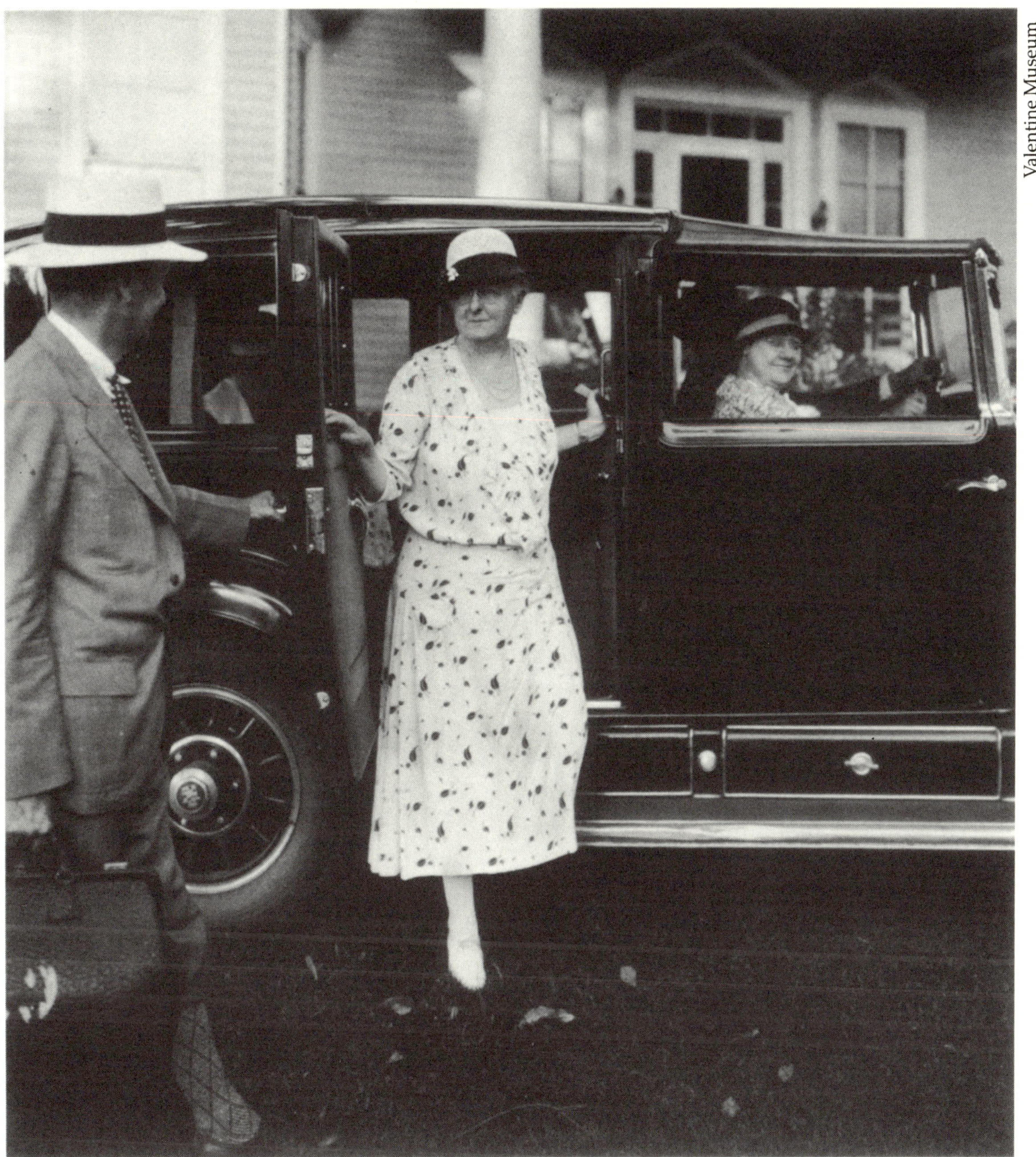

Valentine Museum

Miss Natalie J. Curtis became superintendent of Sheltering Arms Hospital in 1922. Soon afterward she convinced her friend, Miss Hazel Hill, to join the nursing staff as assistant superintendent and teacher of nursing students. Together they were a remarkable team in guiding the efficient growth of Sheltering Arms. As superintendent, Miss Curtis showed her remarkable discernment of people when she persuaded Bertha Woody Hobson to enter nurses' training. Mrs. Hobson, a widow, had been a patient at Sheltering Arms for almost a year in 1922. Once she recovered and settled her young son with her parents, Mrs. Hobson entered the Sheltering Arms School of Nursing in 1923. Upon graduation in 1926, she first worked as a floor nurse, then as an operating room nurse, before Miss Curtis appointed her night supervisor, a position she ably filled for twenty-seven years, until her retirement in 1955.

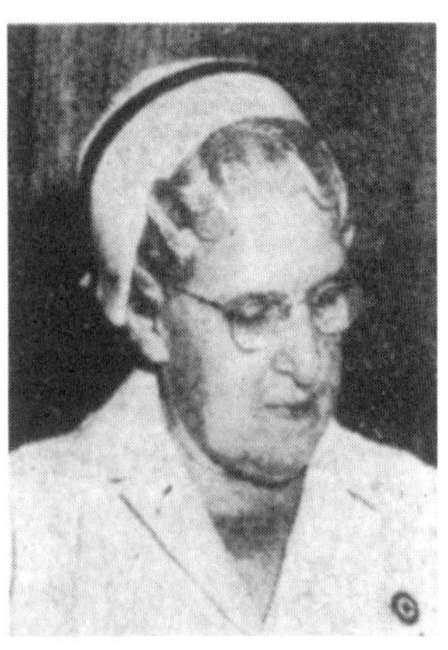

Mrs. Bertha Hobson, associated with Sheltering Arms from 1923 to 1955—first as a patient, then as a student nurse, and finally as the responsible night supervisor.

Right: 1926 graduating class of the Sheltering Arms School of Nursing: Bertha Hobson, center front row; Hazel Hill, third from left, back row; Natalie Curtis, third from right, back row; Tommy Curtis in front.

Miss Curtis' staff continued to be strengthened in the late 1920s by the appointment of Miss Laura Vietor as head nurse. She was an experienced nurse with training in pharmacology at Johns Hopkins and she made a significant contribution during nearly forty years she devoted to Sheltering Arms.

Hard decisions and added responsibility for Sheltering Arms were brought on by the worldwide financial depression that followed the stock market crash of 1929. When hungry neighborhood children began to wait outside the Hospital kitchen for food, members of the executive board decided to donate food to them and a hot meal was served daily at the back door by the cook, Mrs. Agnes Turpin. There were hundreds of names on the waiting list for admission to the Hospital, including many who had never before needed financial help. The Hospital now furnished free bed and board to a number of registered nurses who were unable to find employment, and as many as possible were added to the payroll at $35 per month.

Also during the Depression several students from the Medical College of Virginia offered help around the Hospital in return for a free meal or a cot for the night. One sympathetic board member of Sheltering Arms rounded up clothes and book money for a certain young man who had endeared himself to

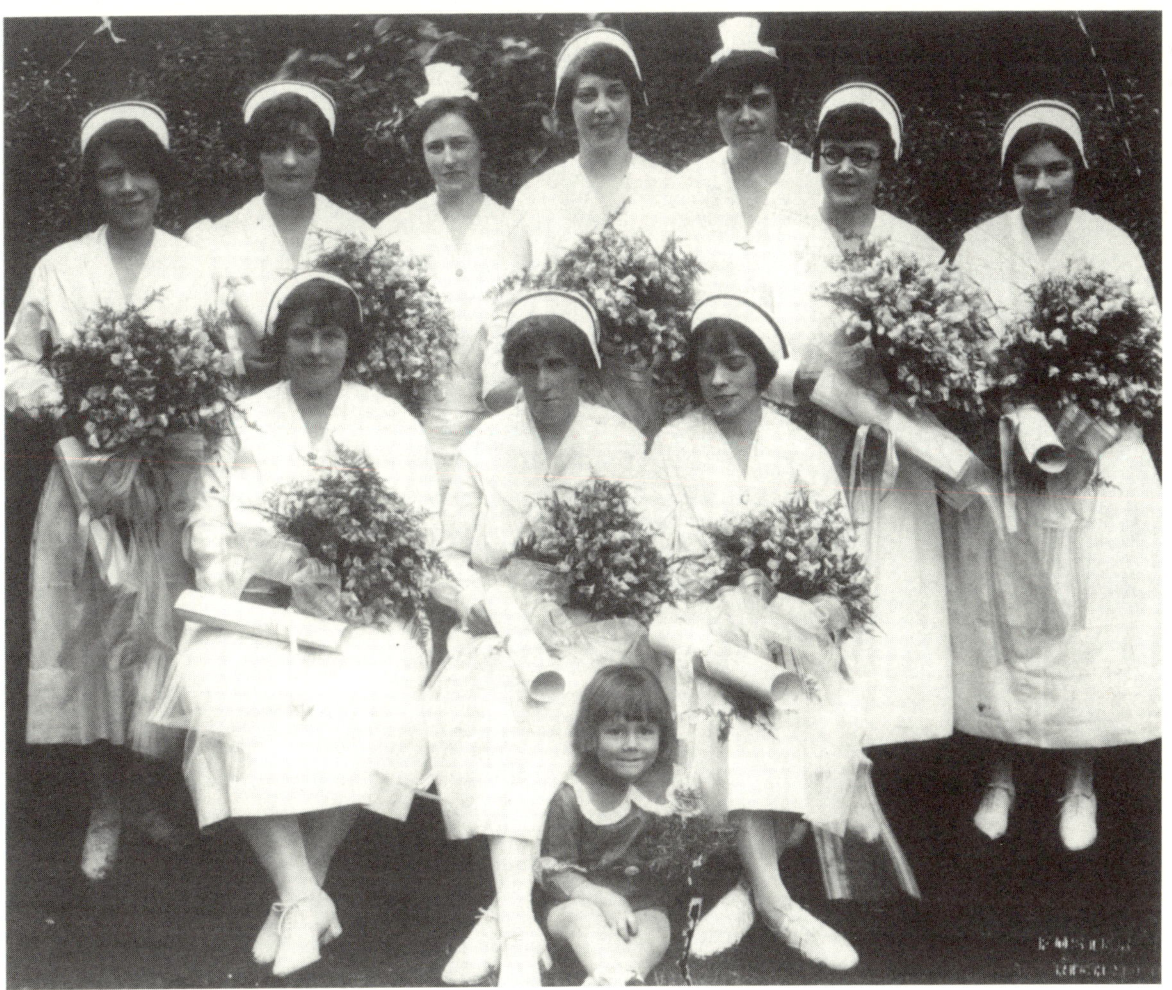
Foster Studio

the Hospital's staff by taking on many middle-of-the-night chores. He later became a psychiatrist and returned to Sheltering Arms to repay the "loan." The board member refused to accept repayment, explaining that she had begged and borrowed it from many sources. In recognition of her generosity, a fund to help medical students was established at the Medical College of Virginia during the 1930s in honor of that generous board member, Mrs. Pauline L. Thalhimer.

During those difficult years Miss Curtis, the Hospital's revered superintendent, found many ways to stretch a penny: the Blackburn bedding company donated mattress ticking, and she used it to make aprons and bedpan covers. She also had old rubber surgical gloves cut into narrow strips to make rubber bands and put patients to useful tasks, too, like cutting up sponges to be sterilized for use in the operating room.

Mrs. George T. King, Hospital treasurer, reported with obvious delight in 1934 that she had been able to pay all the February bills in February, "which has not happened in years!"

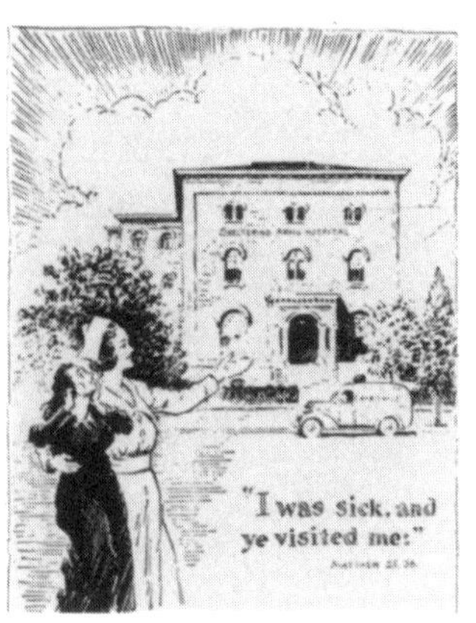

Fiftieth Anniversary Founders Day sketch for the Richmond Times-Dispatch by Fred O. Seibel.

Through the years thousands of people who could not afford to be sick were returned to health by treatment received at Sheltering Arms, and thousands of babies were born there. Operations at Sheltering Arms saved sight, skin grafts helped heal burns, cleft palates and club feet were corrected, and broken bones mended. The contributions of the hundred or more physicians who freely gave their service at Sheltering Arms made it possible to bring patients into the healing home on East Clay Street.

Others gave of themselves in different ways. Miss Mary Boyd (later Mrs. James A. Jones), a young graduate student at the Presbyterian School of Christian Education in 1932 and 1933, remembers catching the bus from Northside to go downtown to read stories to patients at Sheltering Arms. Both children and adults loved her thoughtful ministrations.

In those difficult Depression years, even more attention was paid to saving money. A practical King's Daughter, Mrs. Bernard L. Reams, collected day-old bread from the bakeries and delivered it to Sheltering Arms, while her husband, a country doctor, brought cheer to Miss Curtis and the Hospital by supplying flowers from his garden whenever he came in to see his patients.

The story of Mattie Knapp typifies the boundless love of the people at Sheltering Arms. In the 1920s Mattie had come from the Methodist orphanage to Sheltering Arms, where she was eager to be trained as a nurse. Unfortunately, she contracted the flu, which led to pneumonia, then emphysema, then severe back problems. Mattie was permanently crippled and unable to continue her training. The board "adopted" Mattie as a "ward of Sheltering Arms," and she lived there until 1967.

Miss Curtis found necessary work for Mattie to do: she manned the front desk and answered the telephone for many years, as well as personally acknowledging the numerous non-cash gifts. Mattie utterly loved Sheltering Arms and gladly did anything she could for the Hospital.

For years the doctors worked at Sheltering Arms with the bare necessities, often bringing their own surgical instruments from their own hospitals to use at Sheltering Arms. X-rays had to be taken elsewhere to be read by radiologists who volunteered their services. Therefore, the gift of an x-ray machine in 1939 was a great boon to the medical staff. This machine was the gift of a civic organization known as Sertoma (an acronym for SERvice TO MAnkind) that became active at Sheltering Arms in the late 1930s. The same group also donated equipment for the dental clinic.

During these decades, the Hospital's services continued to expand, and its physical plant grew to accommodate them. In addition to the Grant House, Sheltering Arms acquired all the buildings on the north side of the 1000 block of East Clay and three small houses nearby on Tenth Street. Three buildings east

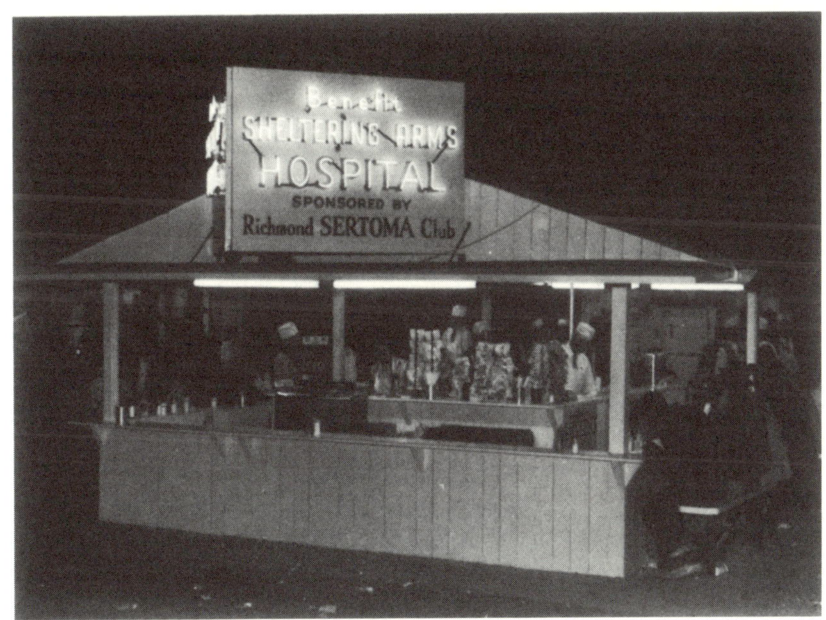

For several decades the Sertoma club ran a food booth at the State Fair for the benefit of Sheltering Arms.

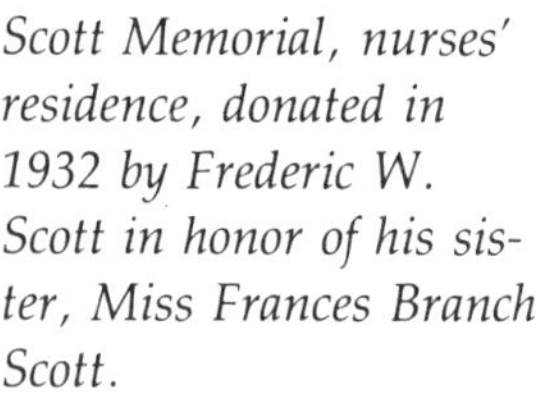

Scott Memorial, nurses' residence, donated in 1932 by Frederic W. Scott in honor of his sister, Miss Frances Branch Scott.

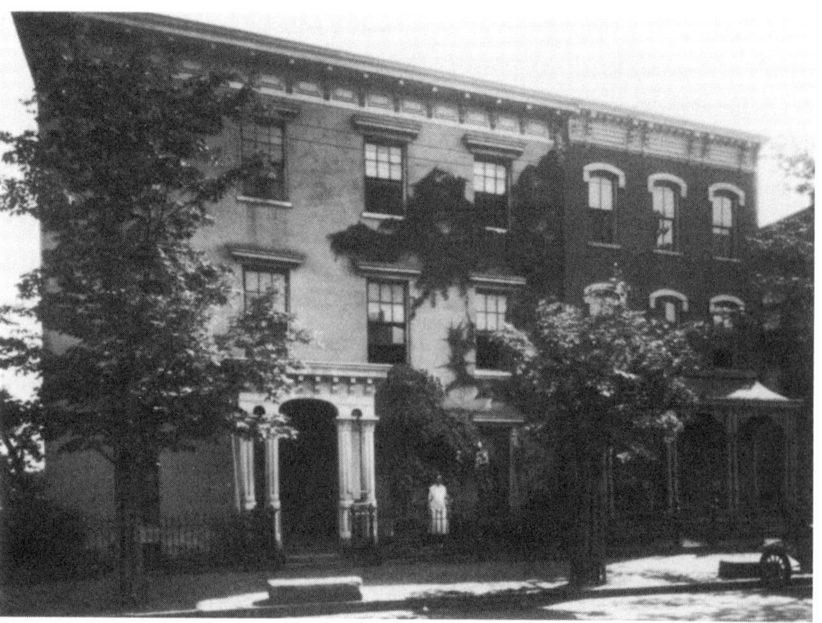

Virginia Historical Society

of the Hospital were the gift of the Reverend John Garlick Scott and his sister, Mrs. Emma Scott Taylor, while an anonymous donor gave the houses on Tenth Street. The buildings on Clay were used as nurses' residences.

The Benjamin Watkins Leigh House on the corner of Tenth and Clay was presented to the Hospital by Frederic W. Scott in 1932. This handsome building, which was erected in 1817, became known as the Scott Memorial and was used as a nurses' home. Miss Curtis and her adopted son Tommy, Miss Hazel Hill, and Mattie Knapp all resided there along with the nurses and nursing students.

One of the nurses who chose to practice at Sheltering Arms for her entire career was Elizabeth Dunn Heubi. Trained under Miss Curtis and Miss Hill and graduated in the last class of the nursing school, in 1934, Mrs. Heubi devoted her professional life to Sheltering Arms, taking time out only to bear two daughters.

Sheltering Arms survived the hard times of the Depression only to face other equally challenging hardships. In 1937 a shortage of nurses forced Miss Curtis to start a training school for licensed practical nurses, in cooperation with Virginia Hospital. By 1940, the trying times of another World War created a shortage of doctors for the civilian population. Many had left Richmond to serve in the 45th General Hospital unit in Italy. During this period patients, too, were scarce for the first time, as employment and wages ran high for the war effort. Yet for Sheltering Arms the year 1941 saw 170 babies born and 1420 patients treated there.

By the end of 1941, a $100,000 addition to the Hospital increased the bed complement from 85 to 103 and added a delivery room to the maternity floor and an isolation room for babies. The three-story addition now formed a connection between Scott Memorial and the Grant House section of the Hospital. No longer did nurses have to dash outside in all sorts of weather to report to Miss Hill's office at 1008 Clay for 6:30 a.m. devotions before going on duty at seven o'clock.

In the aftermath of the Great Depression, national health insurance became a public policy issue. But Sheltering Arms Hospital was already dealing with inequity in health service by giving free care, thanks to the generosity of private citizens who helped to pay for those in need of hospitalization.

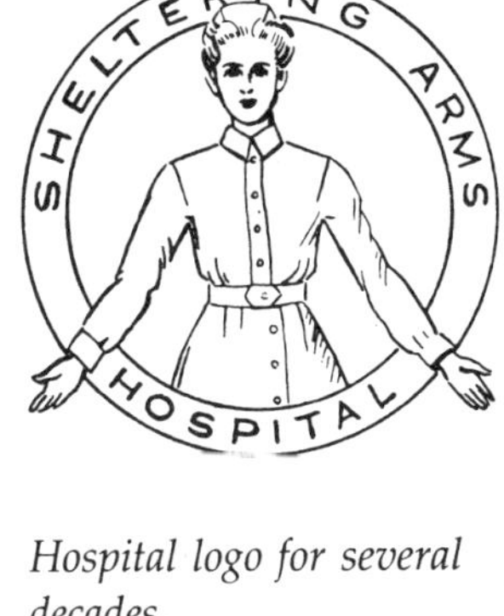

Hospital logo for several decades.

Lower: Baby nursery–a favorite duty of Sheltering Arms nurses.

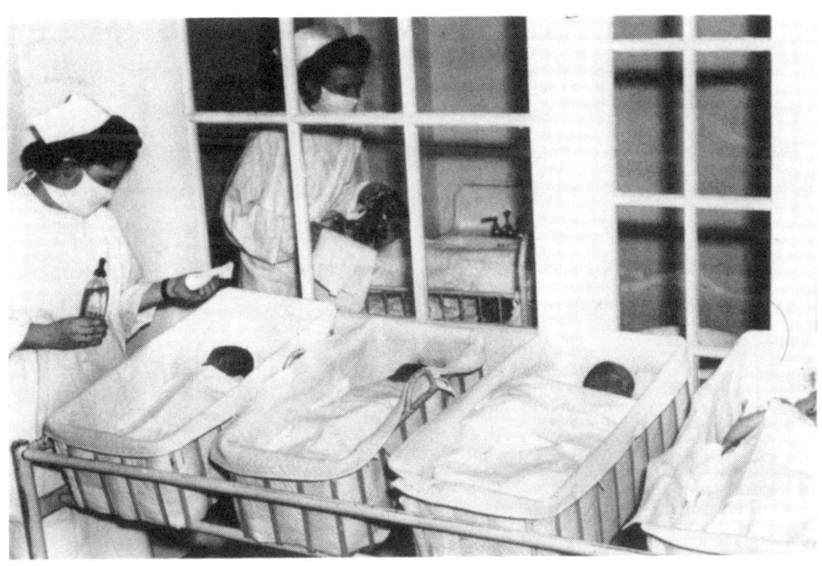

Through the turbulent times of the 1940s, the loyal support of many groups and individuals was responsible in large measure for the steadiness of the ship. The Hospital's devoted volunteers and board members were steadfast. Mrs. Louise Price was a quiet, vital force behind the volunteer effort. She organized the coverage, 365 days a year, of the front desk at 1008 East Clay. At that desk, all traffic in and out the front door was controlled, and all telephone calls from outside the Hospital and in-house lines were thoughtfully directed by the volunteer on duty. Elizabeth Walton, the volunteer with longest service at Sheltering Arms, began her work under Mrs. Price and has continued for almost forty years.

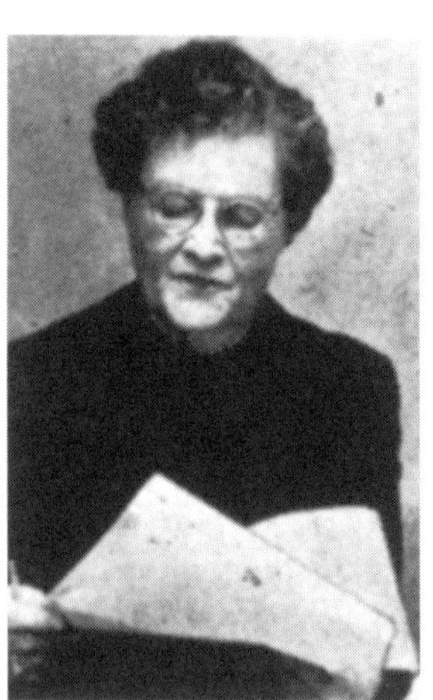

Mrs. Louise Crutchfield Price, conscientious chairman of volunteers at Sheltering Arms for 20 years.

As Mesdames Frazier, Williams, McElroy, and Michaux presided at General Board meetings during the 1950s, who can ever forget seeing the two stalwart King's Daughters leaders—Mrs. Archie McCalley of Cup of Cold Water Circle and Mrs. Roy Caudle of Hope Circle—sitting *ex cathedra* in the tall boardroom chairs up front?

Tales abound of help given to support the work of Sheltering Arms. Many King's Daughters were veritable linchpins in the daily provision of goods and services. Mrs. Sadie Jacobs vowed that her husband always planted his vegetable garden in the pattern of "one row for the family, one row for Sheltering Arms." In those days people from far and near brought hampers of vegetables to the Hospital. Mrs. Walter Reid of Health Circle said she "tried to do the little things" for Sheltering Arms. Working in the sewing room of the old Hospital, she patched the sheets and made "johnnie coats" for the nurses out of old white shirts.

Sometime after World War II the Junior Board was reactivated, bringing more young women volunteers into the life of the Hospital.

The post-war economic boom hit Richmond, and one side effect was the installation of air conditioning in shops and offices. Sheltering Arms did not enjoy the luxury of air conditioning, but every effort was made to make the patients comfortable.

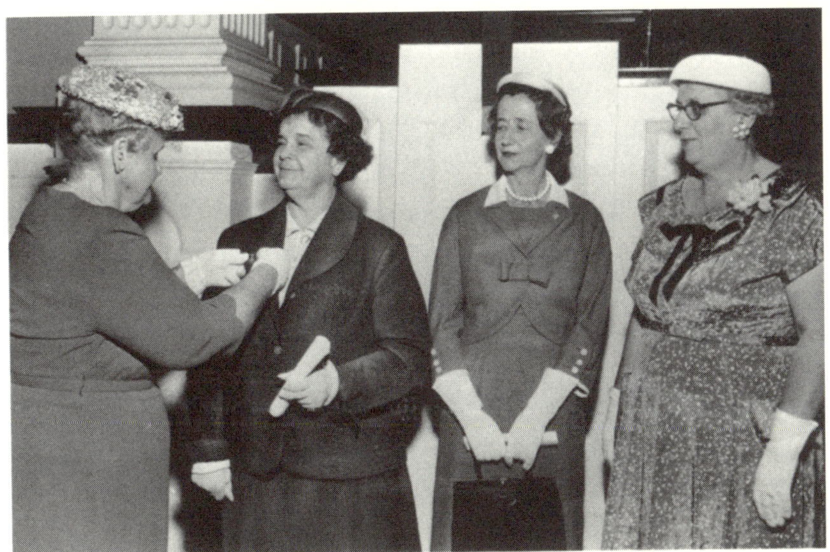

Upper: King's Daughters' recognition of Mrs. Roy Caudle's service. Mrs. Archie McCalley, Mrs. Caudle, Mrs. John L. McElroy, Mrs. Earle Brown, left to right.

Lower: Mrs. Edward C. Anderson, president of the Board of Managers, 1948-1950, inspecting donated canned goods.

Devastating as it must have seemed at the time, the leading nurses retired in quick succession: Miss Curtis and Miss Hill on December 31, 1954; Mrs. Hobson, the night supervisor, in 1955; and Miss Vietor, head nurse, in 1955. For a short period, Miss Evelyn Heath became superintendent. From 1958 to 1965 Mrs. Heubi was the director of nursing and Mrs. Nancy Murray, the assistant director.

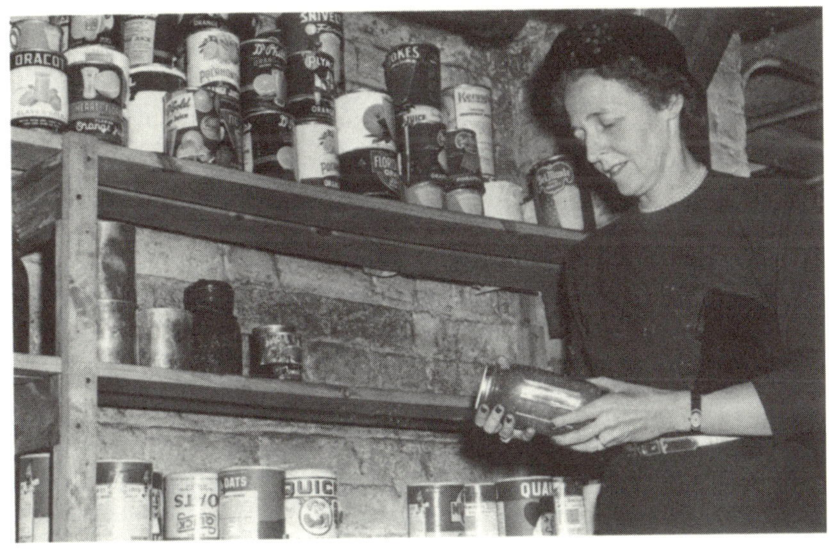

The women's board recognized the need for professionally trained administrators, and in 1957 hired its first business manager. In 1958 they also chose Samuel Waddell to serve as the Hospital's first administrator. Joseph Ahlschier, the second professional administrator, will be remembered for his good sense in hiring young Nancy Mann Barret in September 1961 to assist in the office. Peter Lambert and Tom McCallie were also administrators for short periods. Volunteers and professionals worked together at Sheltering Arms for the good of the patients and the Hospital. Often the professionals volunteered their time and talent, and the volunteers worked like professionals.

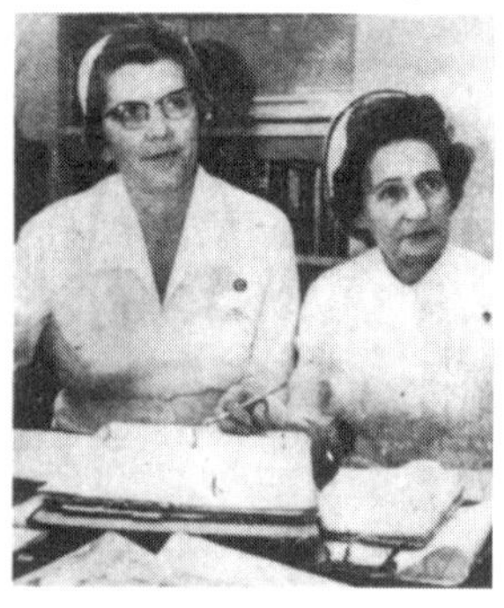

Mrs. Elizabeth Heubi, director, and Mrs. Nancy Murray, assistant director of nursing.

Lower: Two patients helping with meal preparation.

Right: St. Catherine students, Lelia Gibson and Ellen Michaux, sort their Thanksgiving food under the supervision of Mrs. Mary Broyles, dietitian.

Sheltering Arms had been built on donations—gifts of time, talent, and treasure. The records show such diversified gifts as a ton of slate, 30 deer in season, 30 dozen duck eggs, innumerable jars of home-canned food, baskets of plums, rutabagas, and potatoes, hundreds of garments from the Needlework Guild, and funds from the doctors to paint the operating room and the exterior woodwork of the Hospital. Donations of money had come from all over Virginia: pennies from Sunday School children, dollar bills from former patients, checks for

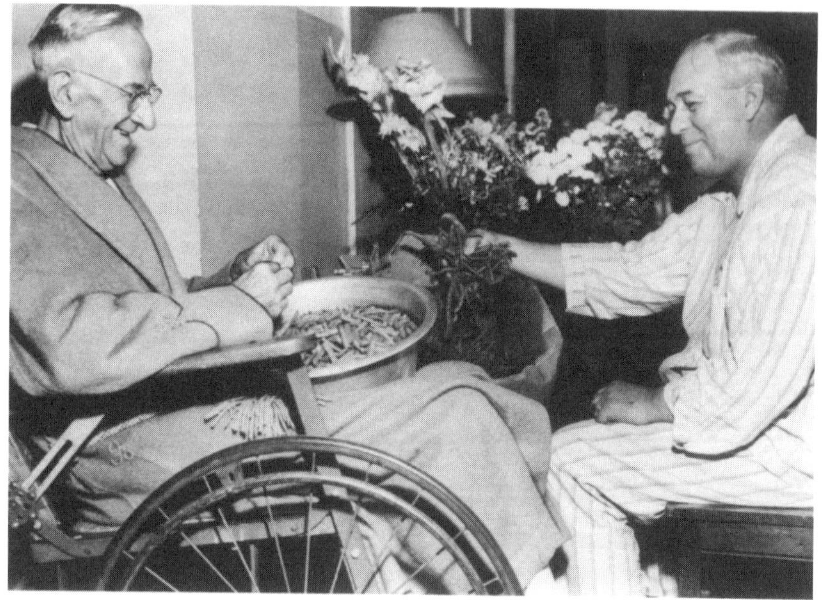

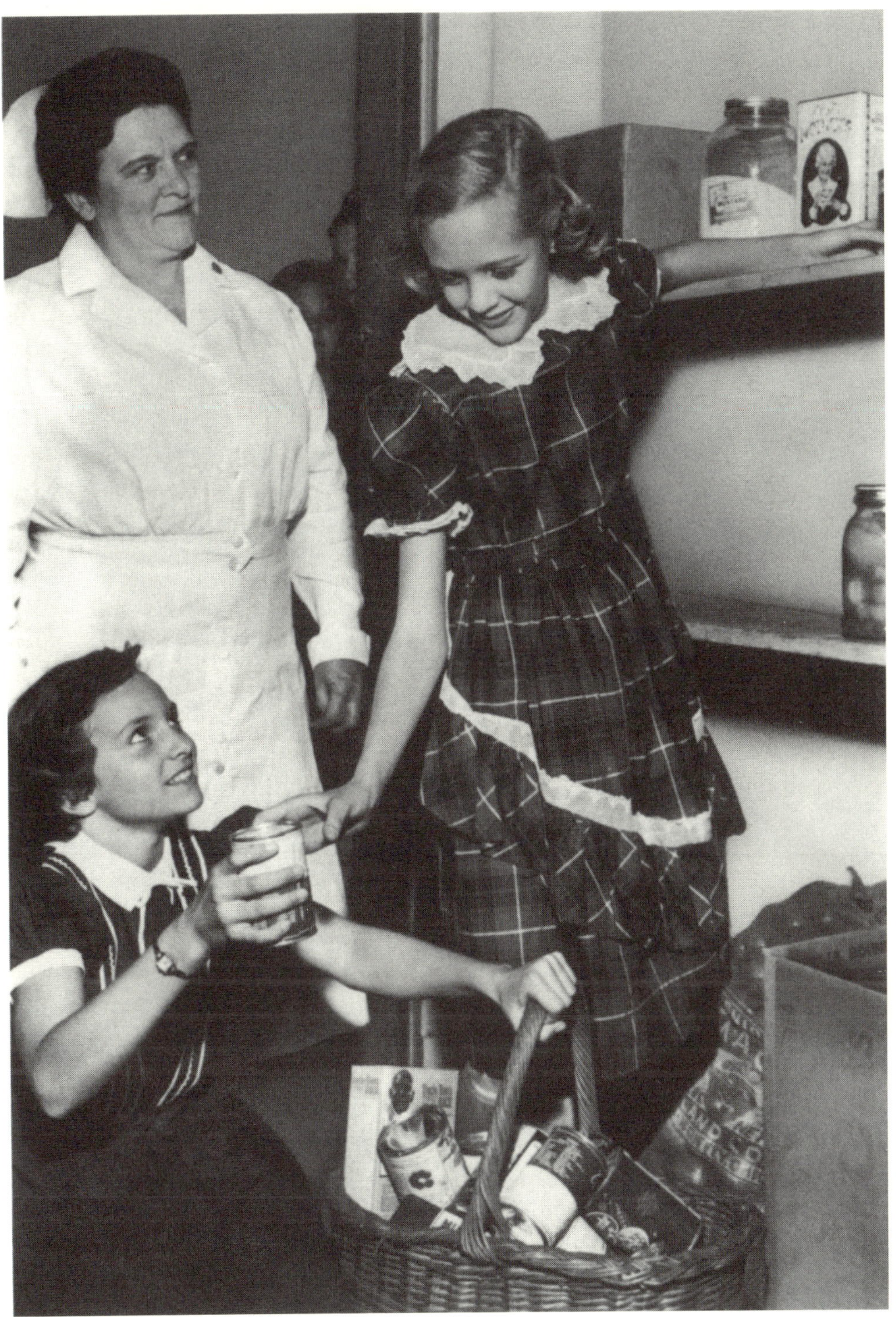

hundreds and thousands of dollars from individuals and groups, and bequests from wills.

By hard work, practiced economy, and the generosity of friends, Sheltering Arms continued to operate. Its nurses were untiring, its doctors unselfish, its staff loving, and its board members and volunteers resolute in offering care to needy people. The spiritual foundations and roots established at Sheltering Arms over the past six decades would not be shaken with the challenge to move to another location.

WE NEED THESE
Cost
TRILENE INHALER FOR
OBSTETRICAL ANESTHESIA
3 DOZEN CUPS AND SAUCERS
3 DOZEN PLATES 3 DOZEN
SOUP BOWLES (VITRIFIED CHINA)
4 DOZEN BATH TOWELS
2 DOZEN BABY SHIRTS

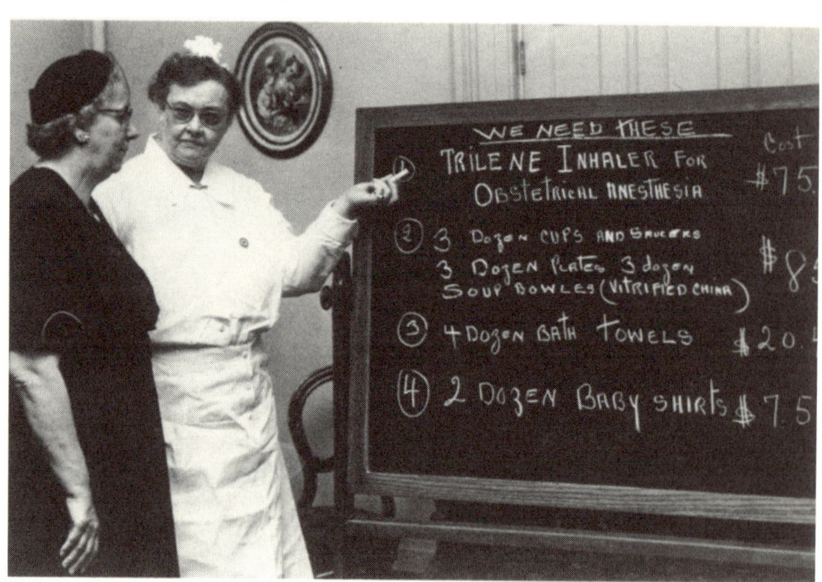

The resourceful superintendent of Sheltering Arms, Miss Natalie Curtis, discusses Hospital needs with Mrs. Earle Brown of The King's Daughters.

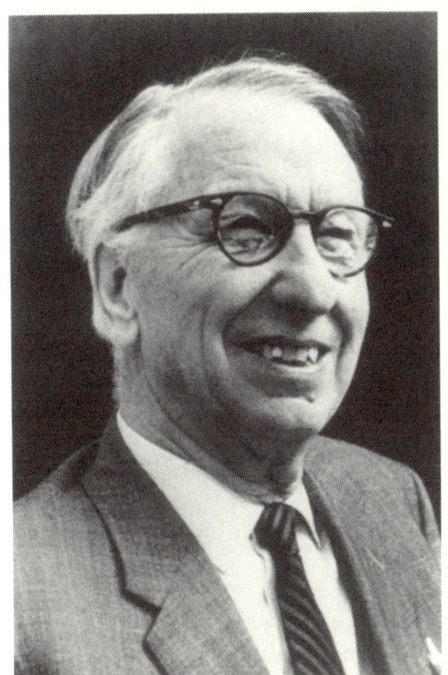

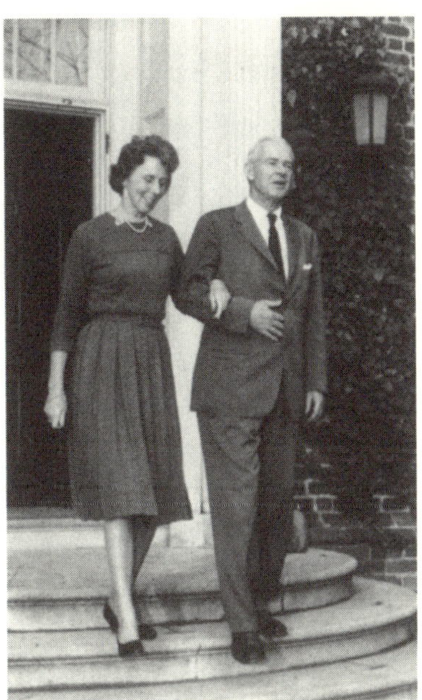

Left: James H. Scott, a devoted trustee of the Hospital, involved for several decades with the Investment Committee and the endowment fund.

Right: Mr. and Mrs. William T. Reed, Jr., active members of the men's and women's boards at the Hospital on Clay Street.

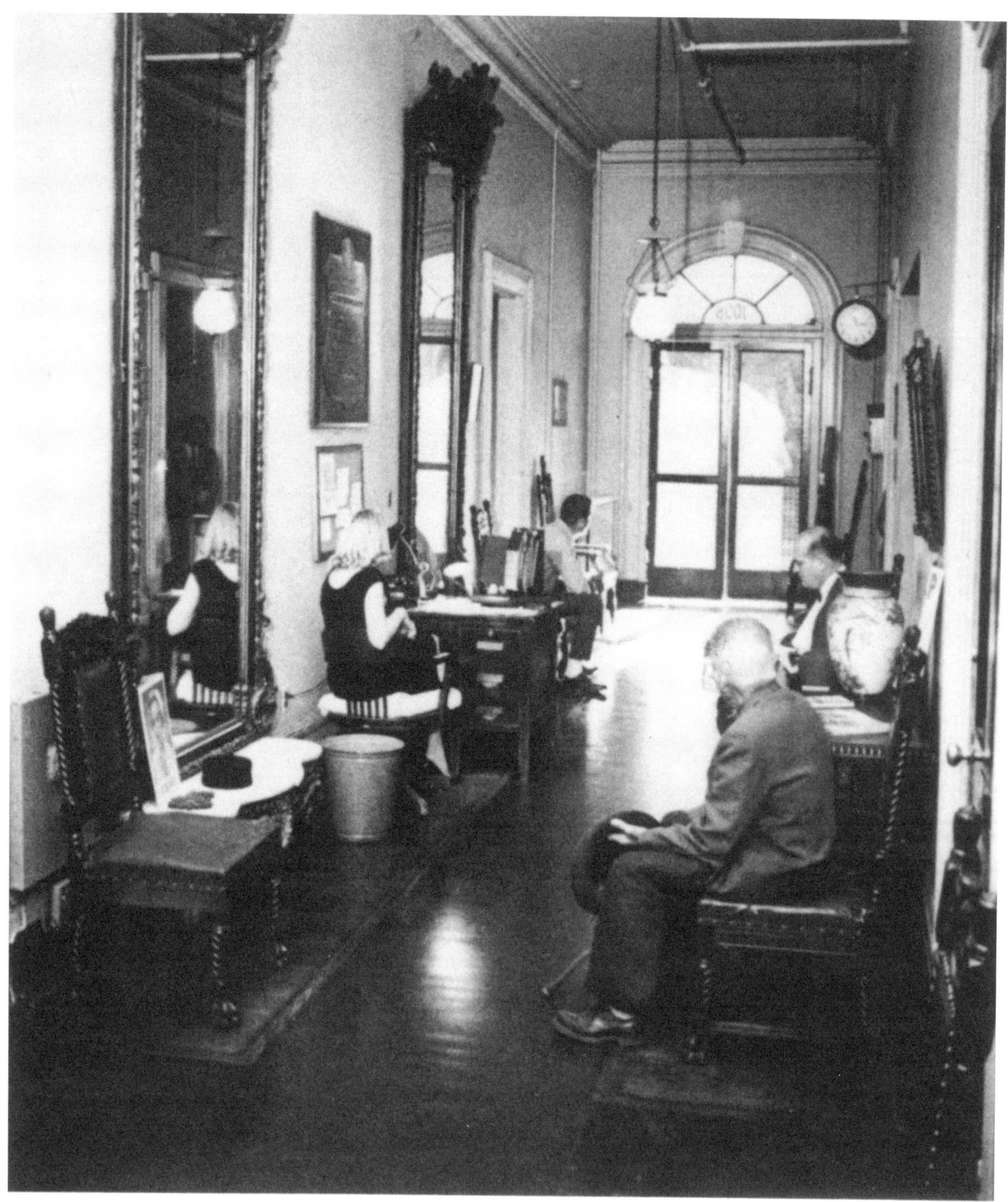

Entrance hallway of the Hospital on Clay Street.

3

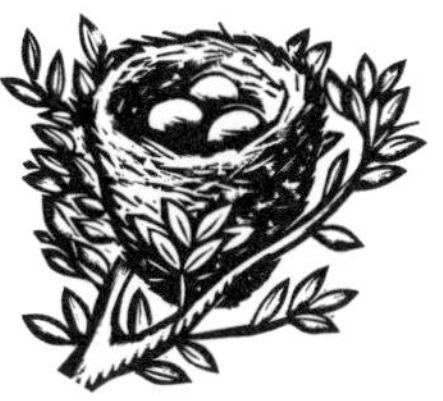

Transplanting the Hospital with a Heart: New Building, New Challenges (1957-1970)

THE YEARS FOLLOWING WORLD WAR II were difficult times for Sheltering Arms. The board of directors felt that the old building had outlived its usefulness; Morton G. Thalhimer, Jr., and William T. Reed, Jr., protectively coaxed the old furnace to continue its duty; and a committee investigated the cost of rebuilding on Clay Street, only to find it prohibitive. The search began for an appropriate location where Sheltering Arms could give service in an economical and efficient manner, yet remain independent to manage its own institution and to control its own resources.

In 1957, Richmond Memorial Hospital opened as a community hospital dedicated to the memory of citizens of Richmond who had fallen in World War II. This new hospital offered the best situation for Sheltering Arms, through an interdependent liaison of two non-profit hospitals. Richmond Memorial could offer in-house services on a contractual basis to Sheltering Arms, which would pay a per diem rate based on cost. Sheltering Arms, on the other hand, would bring with it the good will of the community and its stature as a beloved hospital.

Careful negotiations between Robert Carter, president of the men's board, and Harold Prather, administrator of Richmond Memorial, forged a contract beneficial to both institutions. Sheltering Arms could remain viable and yet independent.

The decision to move and to ally itself with another institution struck a chord in the hearts of those who knew Sheltering Arms. The need to do so was evident, but traumatic for everyone who had served Sheltering Arms for one, two, even three generations in some families. It brought deep sadness to many doctors who felt Sheltering Arms had been the most rewarding part of their practice. And it brought a feeling of confusion to the large corps of nurses who had made Sheltering Arms a "haven of mercy" since 1889. During the years of negotiations Mrs. Thomas F. Wheeldon led the ladies' board in the daily life of the Hospital.

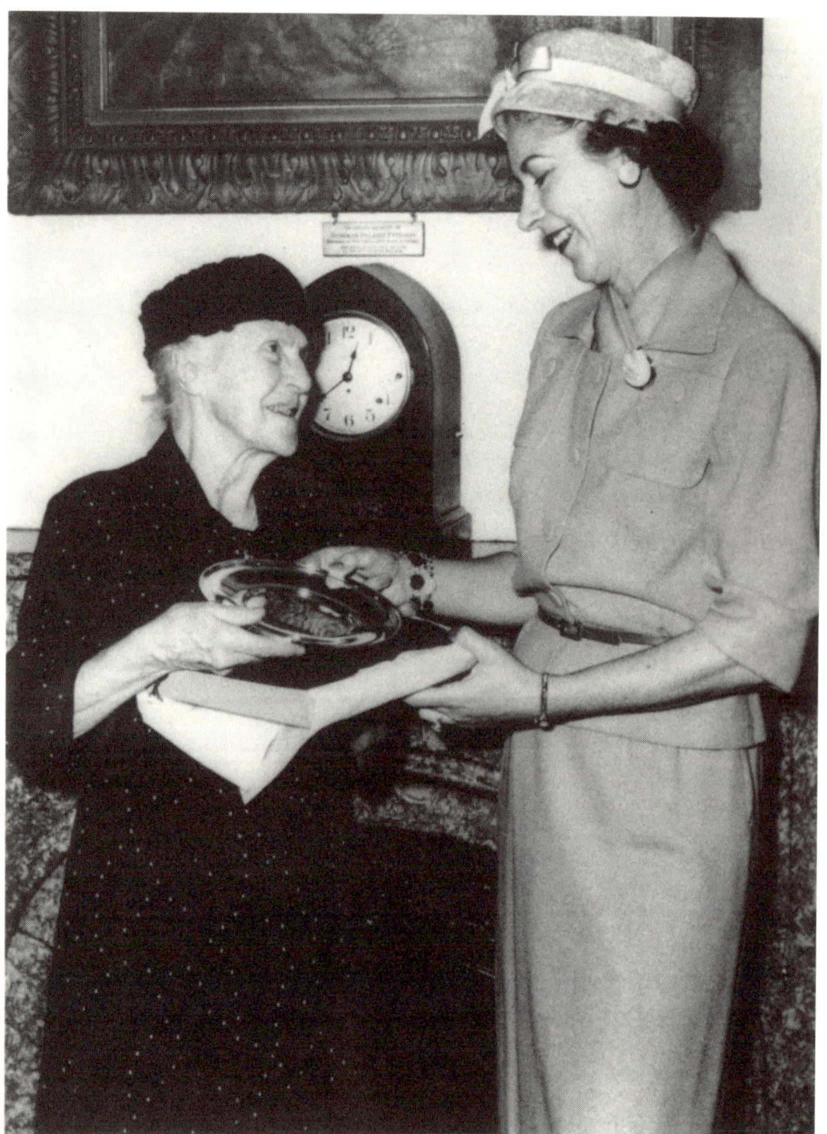

Miss Paula Schulmeister, upon her retirement in 1961, receives a silver plate from board president Mrs. Thomas Wheeldon. She had been medical records librarian for 17 years.

The decision to move was announced to the public by Robert Carter in November 1961. The following year, an agreement was signed for Sheltering Arms to build a new 50-bed hospital on the grounds of Richmond Memorial, the largest of the existing independent hospitals with an available building site and one that was subject to neither individual nor state control.

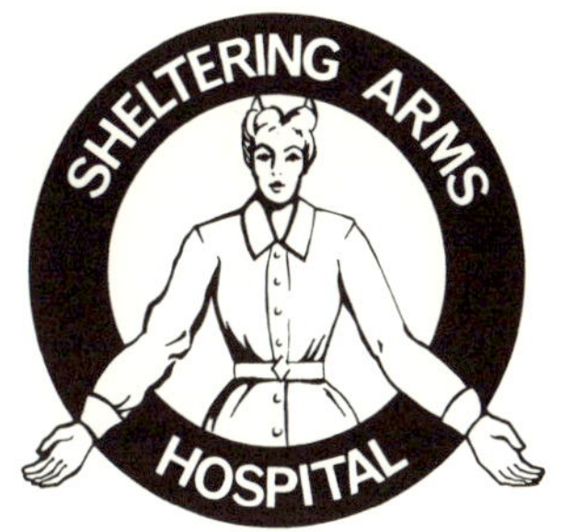

Sheltering Arms logo until 1980.

The new building would cost $1,625,000: 55 percent from federal Hill-Burton funds, 37.5 percent from Sheltering Arms Hospital, and 7.5 percent from Richmond Memorial Hospital. The Building Fund Committee, under S. Buford Scott, felt Sheltering Arms' share would come from the sale of the East Clay property, gifts from interested friends, and from the endowment fund.

On July 17, 1963, groundbreaking for the new hospital was led by Arthur S. Brinkley, Jr., president of the men's board, and little Eda Atkinson Martin, age six, representing four generations of service to the hospital by the Williams family. In November of that same year, the cornerstone was sealed by Morton G. Thalhimer III, age nine, who also represented four generations of faithful workers.

Into that stone went cherished mementoes: the silver cross and motto of The King's Daughters, histories of the Hospital and of the Florence Nightingale Circle, a Donation Day brochure, a copy of prayers said at the groundbreaking, and a list of organizations working for the Hospital.

As the Hospital was moved a few miles to the north, it took with it the prayers, the faith, the love, the friends of four generations, and the assurance that there would be new friends to keep alive the traditions and spiritual legacy of Sheltering Arms.

Of course the entire staff was affected by the decision to move Sheltering Arms to the Northside. The nurses who had given so much of their time and talent to serve Sheltering Arms patients for so many years wondered about their future with the new hospital. Although Richmond Memorial generously

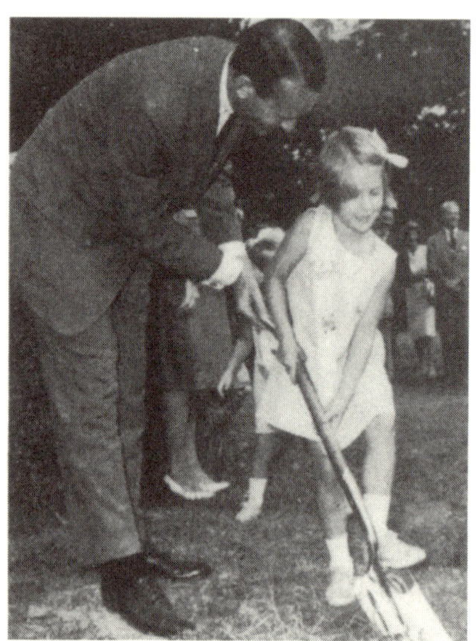

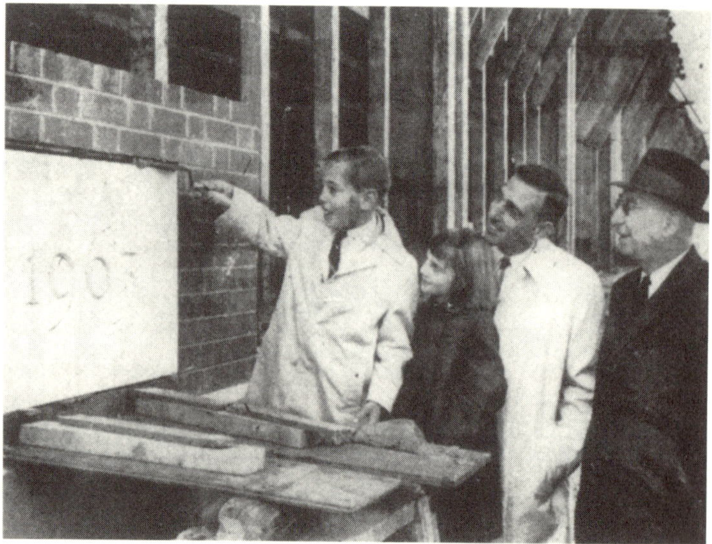

pledged to find employment for every Sheltering Arms employee, only one registered nurse transferred: Mrs. Elizabeth Heubi was to be head nurse, until the position of liaison nurse was created. Virginia Loving transferred to Palmyra Avenue and is still working in the laundry department. Others who moved were Lillian Johnson, medical records; and licensed practical nurses Margaret Dill, Frances Wissler, Earline Vaughan, and Lydell Dowell. Nancy Barret and Sophie Gayle moved to the new executive and finance offices, and Miss Vietor went as a volunteer to oversee the drug room. The beloved orderly Foster Berry moved to Palmyra Avenue after nearly thirty years on Clay Street, as did Willie Brown, a porter.

How could a tradition such as Sheltering Arms be transplanted without losing its spirit? The Board of Managers set itself to the task, and the move was accomplished. Mrs. Henry Bullock (Pat) efficiently organized the dispersal of all useful items. Mrs. William H. Emory, Jr. (Emma Gray) recalls the fruitless effort to give away the old hospital beds, known as "cots," which were quite outdated by 1964. Mrs. George H. Flowers, Jr. (Mary Frances), president of the Board of Managers, praised the spirit of these women: to be flexible yet to practice frugality, as always.

Volunteers carried the brass plaques off the old hospital's doors and walls to the new hospital as a continuing memorial to past donors. Members of the board carried the revered portraits of founding members, while others helped to move the board room's lovely Victorian furniture. Working together, ever mindful of its beginnings, the people of Sheltering Arms Hospital created a new home with old traditions. The spirit of dedication to care for the needy was transplanted to a beautiful, new, and efficient setting. There were fifty-three beds. With an eye for taste and discretion, Mrs. William G. Reynolds (Mary) worked with Thalhimers department store to create a fitting interior decor.

Left: The fourth generation of two families associated with Sheltering Arms: Eda Martin, great granddaughter of Alice Taylor Williams, assists board president Arthur S. Brinkley, Jr., with groundbreaking for the Hospital on Palmyra, and Morton G. Thalhimer III, with his sister, father, and grandfather, seals the cornerstone.

With the inspiring words of Dr. Theodore F. Adams, the new Sheltering Arms building was dedicated on January 19, 1965. Dr. Ariel L. Goldburg and the Most Reverend John J. Russell assisted in the ceremony. By the first of February all the patients were moved from Clay Street to Palmyra Avenue.

The brick building on Palmyra Avenue, which faced north on Lamont Street, now greeted visitors and patients, its "honored guests," through two-story glass panels. Above the doorway was inscribed Mrs. George T. King's chosen verse, "Behold what God hath wrought."

The grounds, designed by Charles Gillette as a gift to Sheltering Arms, complemented the modern architecture, designed by Baskervill & Sons. The front entrance was enhanced by a lovely marble fountain, the gift of Frank E. Brown, a board member of both Sheltering Arms and Richmond Memorial. The Hospital's outward appearance was quite different from the stately Grant House on Clay Street, but inside, its heart continued to beat with the same willingness to help people in need.

As one entered the front door of Sheltering Arms, the flurry of activity in the office to the left was generated by the smiling small dynamo, Nancy Barret. Here was the nerve center of the enterprise. Daily telephone contact with referring physicians kept radiating the message of Sheltering Arms out to the Northern Neck, Tidewater, and the mountains of Virginia. Certain general practitioners and internists of decades past still turned to Sheltering Arms for that special element of care, referring their patients to the new hospital.

Here, too, volunteers still served at the reception desk and the switchboard. They escorted patients and answered their needs for everyday items. Yes, and here were Miss Vietor and Katy Robinson in a cubicle designed to be an elevator, carefully putting on shelves the drug samples donated by local doctors and pharmaceutical houses. The life of Sheltering Arms went on; it had to—people without money continued to need hospitalization.

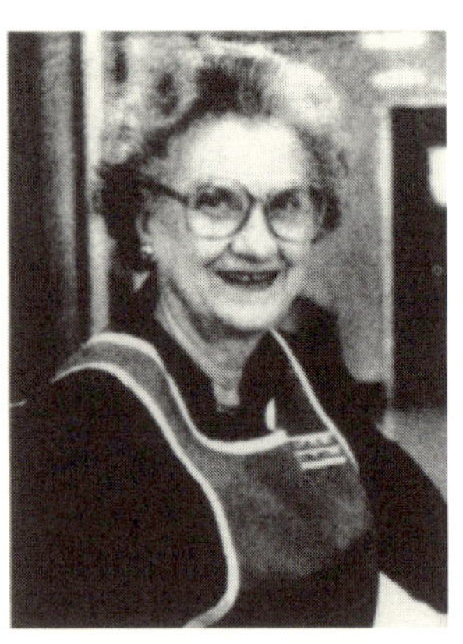

Katy Robinson, a volunteer for many years, covered the telephone desk and assisted Miss Vietor in the drug room.

By arrangement with Richmond Memorial, many of the Hospital's functions were provided by the larger institution at a cost-saving plan. Nursing, the operating room, dietary, housekeeping, maintenance, security, and certain ancillary and administrative services were provided by Richmond Memorial. Sheltering Arms, in turn, paid a per diem rate to Richmond Memorial to cover those services in a contractual arrangement beneficial to both institutions. Actually, from February 1965 to June 1980, Sheltering Arms had only three employees: Nancy Barret, administrative secretary; Elizabeth Heubi, R.N.; and Helen Sterling, financial secretary, who replaced Miss Gayle.

In its new location at 1311 Palmyra Avenue, Sheltering Arms kept its traditional admissions policy, by which patient applications would be reviewed by a committee of the Board of Managers. Admissions would be processed through the Sheltering Arms admitting office. Doctors continued to give their services free of charge to Sheltering Arms patients. All Sheltering Arms funds were held and administered by its own board of directors. All donations of drugs and supplies were credited to Sheltering Arms.

Mr. Harold Prather, who had come from Tennessee to administer Richmond Memorial when it opened in 1957, also took on the duties of administrator of Sheltering Arms. He graciously welcomed Sheltering Arms, fully cognizant of his responsibility to help it survive. Meeting almost daily with Mary Frances Flowers, who zealously guarded the obligation to provide the finest service to Sheltering Arms patients, Mr.

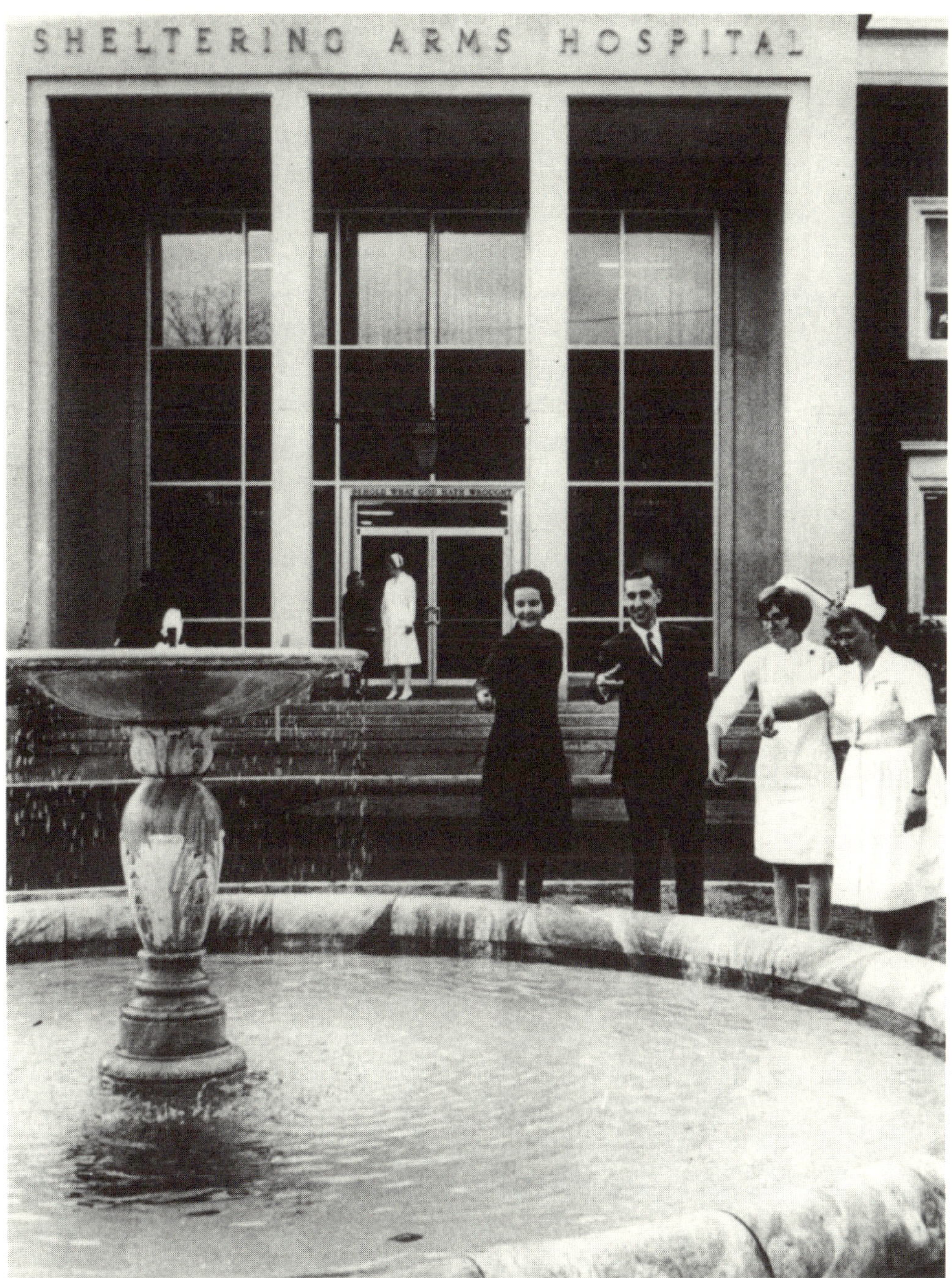

In celebration of the 1966 Donation Day, presidents Emma Gray Emory (Board of Managers) and Morton G. Thalhimer, Jr. (Board of Directors), and nurses Lynda Sharp and Madeline Flournoy, throw coins in the new fountain, a gift of Frank E. Brown.

Prather successfully assisted Sheltering Arms in its period of adjustment.

At first, medical care at Sheltering Arms was under the direction of Dr. Barry Decker, then Dr. I. Norman Sporn, and then Dr. Jerome Smith. Eventually, in 1971, Dr. William Anderson, a full-time employee of Richmond Memorial, became the director of the medical and surgical staff. The old tradition, whereby physicians donated their services to Sheltering Arms, continued, and Sheltering Arms did not pay for this "professional component." In this same era of good will and generous intentions, however, Richmond Memorial's policies governing physicians, and the new federal laws regulating care for the elderly and the indigent, had an effect on Sheltering Arms' relationships with local doctors. Referring physicians could not follow their patients as freely, and reimbursement for physicians' services became mandatory, a notion foreign to the many doctors who had donated their services to Sheltering Arms for almost eighty years.

With the advent of Medicare in 1965 and Medicaid in 1970, hospital care for elderly and some indigent patients could be reimbursed by the government. But many typical Sheltering

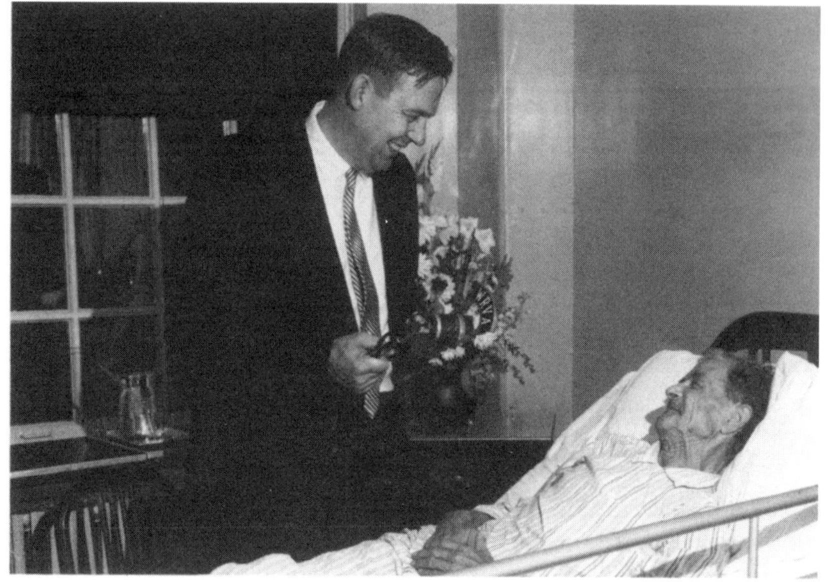

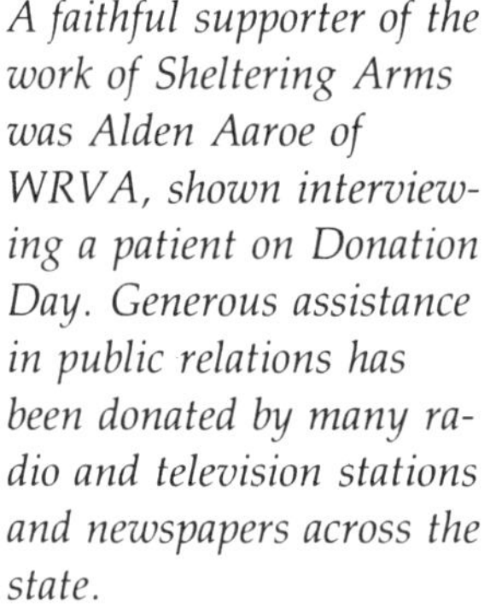
A faithful supporter of the work of Sheltering Arms was Alden Aaroe of WRVA, shown interviewing a patient on Donation Day. Generous assistance in public relations has been donated by many radio and television stations and newspapers across the state.

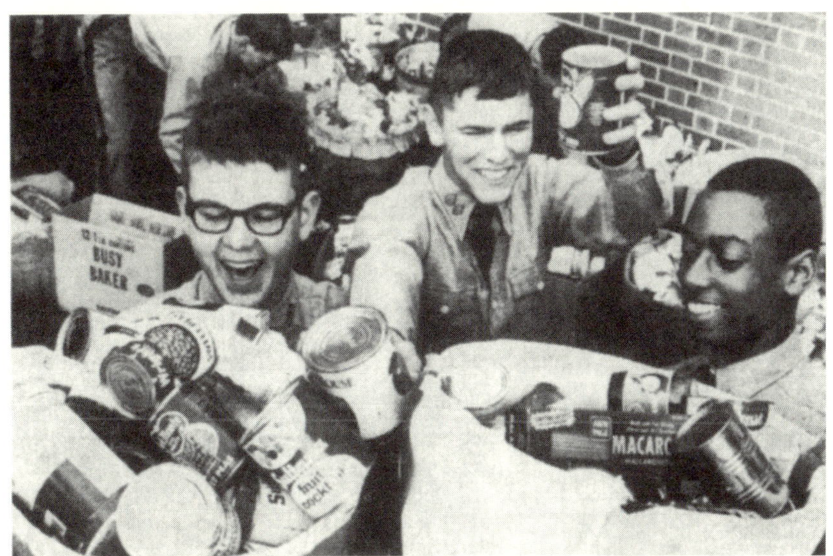

Boys in the John Marshall High School Cadet Corps help unload eleven truck-loads of food donations to the Hospital.

Arms patients did not qualify for government programs because they did not meet eligibility requirements. Sheltering Arms underwrote their care. Although bills were sent to private and government carriers, no Sheltering Arms patient was ever sent a bill.

Admission to Sheltering Arms had one requirement: the donation of a pint of blood by the patient or his family. Most people willingly complied, giving more than one pint even if they did not have surgery themselves. A careful record was kept by Margaret Hunter, a loyal King's Daughter volunteer, who reported monthly to the Board of Managers and was responsible to the Richmond Memorial Blood Bank.

Otherwise, the admission criteria developed by the board made Sheltering Arms' care available to any Virginian regardless of his or her ability to pay. For the first time, this also included black patients. Children were placed in the pediatric unit of Richmond Memorial Hospital, where Sheltering Arms underwrote the per diem cost and doctors donated their services. Most pediatric patients with ear, nose and throat problems were transferred to Richmond Eye Hospital, where they were also cared for without charge.

Sheltering Arms was an acute care hospital with its services limited to medical and surgical cases, no obstetrics. Sheltering Arms did not admit long-term cases, for it was neither a nursing home nor a psychiatric institution. The philosophy was to accept normally self-supporting individuals who were facing a medical crisis without the funds to pay for hospitalization. It held steadfast to its original goal, to help the medically indigent population of Virginia and return them to productive lives in home, school, job, or community work.

How was the fee paid? Chiefly by donations from individuals and groups who supported the Hospital, and by income from the endowment fund. Over the years there was an increasing amount paid by a third party, namely private health insurance companies and Medicare.

The federal government aided the building of many hospitals in the 1960s and 1970s and Sheltering Arms availed itself of these funds to complete its building fund for the new hospital. Although the Building Fund Committee had produced $731,250 for the new hospital, $893,750 more was lent by the federal government in Hill-Burton funds to complete the job. The Hill-Burton Act of Congress stipulated that recipient hospitals must reciprocate by doing charity work equal to the value of the Hill-Burton funds. To be sure, Sheltering Arms did great charity work, but all its patients did not necessarily qualify as charity patients, because they might own their means of livelihood, such as a paint truck, an oyster boat, a taxicab, or a small piece of land, and therefore not meet the government definition of "charity." It was a good many years before Sheltering Arms could fulfill its obligation to the federal Department of Health, Education and Welfare. Margaret Hunter, first as a volunteer and then as a staff member, assiduously kept the records to prove a patient's need for charity care, then justified it in the medical records to HEW, until all $893,750 had been accounted for by Sheltering Arms for charity patients.

Patients often had special needs, such as toothbrushes, bathrobes, warm sweaters, or taxi fare to the Hospital. Mrs. Heubi helped meet them. With her beatific smile and crisp white uniform, she beamed hope and confidence into the patients and their anxious families. As liaison nurse, she communicated simply and eloquently the human condition and the needs of the patients to the lay Board of Managers. Her perceptive liaison encouraged a ready willingness on the part of the volunteer board to spare no effort for the patients' benefit. Both staff and volunteers continued to make each patient feel like an "honored guest" at Sheltering Arms.

The organization of Sheltering Arms continued to include the Board of Directors, all men, who had fiduciary responsibilities; the Board of Managers, all women, who managed the daily

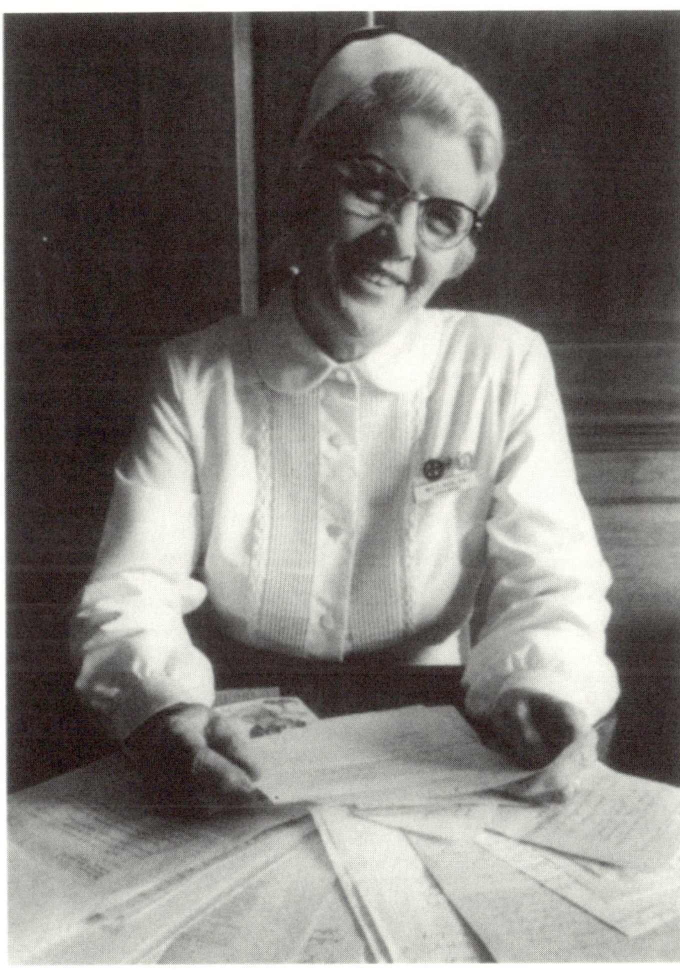

Elizabeth Heubi, Liaison Nurse at the new hospital, epitomized the deep caring for every patient which was synonymous with the name of Sheltering Arms.

operations of the Hospital; the Junior Board, which acted as a major fund raising group and a source of volunteer help; and the General Board, composed of interested groups and individuals who worked for the Hospital, representing The King's Daughters and other mainstays of Sheltering Arms' community support.

In 1965 Buford Scott, a former board president, gave to Sheltering Arms a house across the street, at 1400 Palmyra Avenue, to be used as nurses' quarters. As before, on Clay Street, the building was called Scott Residence. The Florence Nightingale Circle graciously assumed the responsibility of its decorating and maintenance, hiring a yardman and a housekeeper. The Nightingales wanted to keep the nurses happy, responding to their needs in many ways. The president of the Nightingales, an ex-officio member of the Hospital's Board of Managers, made monthly reports on Scott Residence. By 1973, however, few nurses needed living quarters, so the board advised that the Scott Residence be sold.

The "hospital with a heart" had survived the transplant to its new home and had met the challenges of the past decade. It now stood poised on the brink of new challenges and new horizons.

4

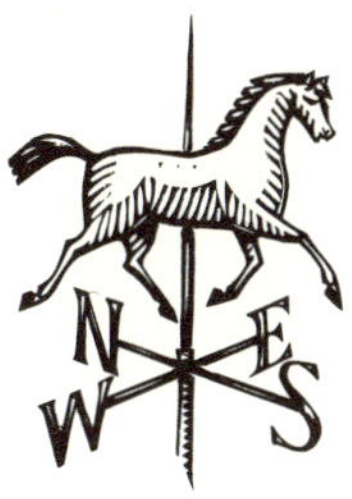

A Vision for the Future: the Change to Rehabilitation Services (1970-1981)

SUBTLE CHANGE WAS OCCURRING in the early seventies: the number of patients referred for acute inpatient care was declining. At the same time, however, outpatient visits to the clinics rapidly increased. The majority of Sheltering Arms patients came from shorter distances, for instance, 75 percent from the greater Richmond area in 1973-74. In 1961 it had made good financial sense to join Richmond Memorial and to purchase services from the larger hospital at cost. But being physically attached to another hospital required constant accommodations between both partners. By 1974 the boards of Sheltering Arms proposed to lease its increasing number of empty beds to Richmond Memorial at a per diem rate. This arrangement was generally a good use of its space, but sometimes led to problems with nursing coverage. Eventually, the Sheltering Arms Board of Managers felt there must be a better solution for the problem of empty beds and the use of the facility. And thus Sheltering Arms began in earnest a process of long range planning, though always in consultation with Richmond Memorial.

Behind the relationship between Sheltering Arms and Richmond Memorial Hospitals was the fact that both were non-profit hospitals, neither desiring to derive financial gain from its activities with the other.

The 1970s was an evolutionary decade. Hospitals everywhere were changing in many ways. The United States was overbedded, the medical profession was experiencing strict regulation, and hospitals were seeking methods to deliver health care in more economic ways. The dynamics of "need" and "demand" were accelerating this period of change in hospitals: change in location of services, change by the development of specializations, change in the ability of more patients to afford specialized care through Medicare and Medicaid. All these factors were affecting the census at Sheltering Arms.

It was a difficult time and Sheltering Arms again sought an answer and a means to survive, quietly and peacefully. It did so by virtue of diligent and extensive study, and by holding firmly to its continuing goal, to offer the most needed form of health care to everyone who could benefit, regardless of their ability to pay.

With a feeling of grave responsibility the boards of Sheltering Arms formed a joint Steering Committee in 1973 to determine whether the Hospital was, in fact, meeting the greatest public need as an acute care general hospital. Made up of both the Board of Managers and the Board of Directors, along with representatives from other support groups, the Steering Committee proceeded to test the waters of change.

William T. Reed III, a leader with foresight, encouraged the boards to study the future possibilities for Sheltering Arms. Dr. Robin MacStravic and his graduate students in the Medical College of Virginia Department of Hospital and Health Administration plumbed the depths of Sheltering Arms' existence and returned with the opinion that Sheltering Arms not only could, but probably should, consider a role change. The Steering Committee evolved into the Long Range Planning Committee. It conferred with members of the medical community and sought expert opinions from health organizations, social welfare agencies, financial institutions, accountants, and planning agencies to see if there was a genuine need for an alternative service at Sheltering Arms.

With singular discernment one of the board members, Dr. Lawrence Prybil, chairman of the Department of Hospital and Health Administration at MCV, established a structured approach to gauge each category of need that the committee identified. Designating the five levels of health care (prevention, primary, secondary, tertiary, and nursing home), the planning committee eventually decided that rehabilitative care (tertiary) seemed to be the most needed in central Virginia. Dr. MacStravic was again called upon to study the feasibility of converting Sheltering Arms to a physical rehabilitation facility. And Dr. Ernest Griffith, chairman of MCV's Department of Rehabilitation Medicine, prepared a proposal for the necessary changes in architecture and program that would be required to convert 1311 Palmyra into a well-integrated rehabilitation facility. A financial feasibility study was complicated, because there was no precedent in Virginia of reimbursement for physical rehabilitation services. This kind of health care would be more expensive than acute care had been, because it was more labor-intensive.

The Hospital anticipated some payment by insurance companies for patients, but in the case of rehabilitation services reimbursement would be retroactive. The boards of Sheltering Arms were willing to take the financial risk in order to offer a service that was desperately needed in central Virginia. They reasoned that since government agencies were not choosing to offer rehabilitation, and private organizations could not afford to provide rehabilitation, Sheltering Arms would fill a real need. After all, for nearly a century the citizens of Virginia had trusted Sheltering Arms to serve those in need, and certainly the need for rehabilitation care did exist. Those victims of stroke, spinal cord injury, neuromuscular disorders, amputation, arthritis,

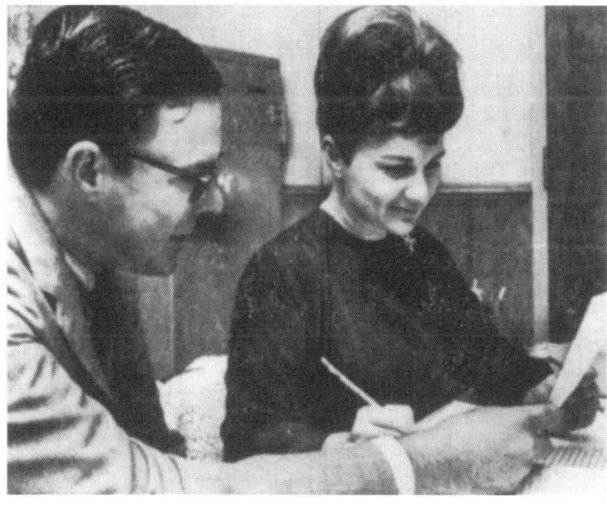

S. Buford Scott and Nancy Barret discuss preparations for Donation Day.

multiple sclerosis, and others, would benefit from a comprehensive rehabilitation facility close to their homes—in Virginia.

Throughout the decision-making process, the department heads of physical therapy and occupational therapy at Richmond Memorial Hospital, Ann Stitzer and Nancy Dawe, were key figures in encouraging Sheltering Arms to consider the merits of a change to physical rehabilitation. John Simpson, administrator of Richmond Memorial after Harold Prather, was supportive of Sheltering Arms' research and feasibility studies for rehabilitation. Mr. Simpson was a positive force as Sheltering Arms carefully studied community and regional health care needs. He offered the opportunity to Sheltering Arms to take over Richmond Memorial Hospital's physical and occupational therapy departments in forming a new Sheltering Arms.

The many studies and field trips by the joint committees of the boards of Sheltering Arms steadily strengthened the resolve to answer the region's need for physical rehabilitation services. Sheltering Arms had maintained 53 acute care beds; in the new plan, 25 of those beds would allow the Hospital to become a comprehensive physical rehabilitation facility.

One of the conscientious leaders of the Hospital through this period was Gilbert Rosenthal. He was forceful in his conviction that third-party carriers would eventually reimburse Sheltering Arms for rehabilitative care, even if assurance could not be prospective. Later, as chairman of the Finance Committee, Mr. Rosenthal was attentive to operations and cost-effective management of Sheltering Arms.

From 1973 to 1979 there were so many meetings to consider the conversion of Sheltering Arms that one committee member, Molly Toms Fitzgerald, claimed her car automatically turned toward the Hospital. Mrs. Fitzgerald, a longtime board member, had financial prudence similar to that of Mrs. George T. King.

In 1961 the decision to move the Hospital had been especially traumatic because it was made without consulting those who were involved in the daily operation of the Hospital.

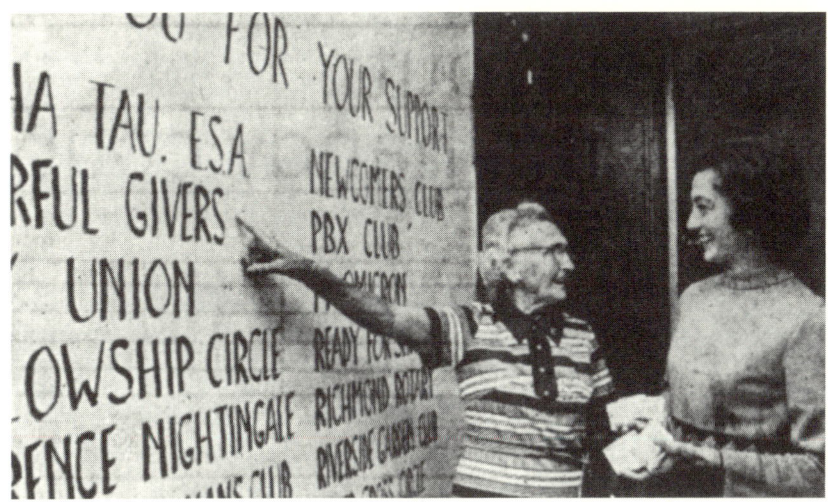

Mrs. Minnie Beadles of the Cheerful Givers Club shares Donation Day enthusiasm with Helen Pinckney (Mrs. C. Cotesworth) of the Junior Board.

As Sheltering Arms faced change again, it was essential that the six-year study process be shared throughout with all concerned, to hear their voices and to ask for their votes on a creative alternative for Sheltering Arms.

Under the strong leadership of Johnnie Lou Terry, president of the Board of Managers, careful consideration was given to keeping all support groups and donors well informed. Once the new organization had been affirmed, Mrs. Terry helped to develop administrative responsibilities, board functions, and new organizational lines of authority.

Mrs. Heubi, the liaison nurse, retired in 1978 after being on duty almost continuously since 1934. In honor of Mrs. Heubi's devotion to her patients, the women's board established the Heubi Fund, to purchase personal equipment that patients could not afford.

It is interesting to note that bequests and donations to Sheltering Arms continued to maintain a high level; in fact, by 1978, the public trust in the Hospital yielded the largest donations to date, both in terms of total amount and in percentage of participation. Wonderfully helpful assistance in public relations was donated by newspapers, television, radio, advertising firms, and others.

Volunteer helpers continued to ask what they could do for the Hospital, and loyal support groups held "imaginary luncheons," Christmas fund raising events, banana split eating contests at Richmond Braves baseball games, demolition derbies, car washes, theatre parties, even trips to the horse races! Ingenuity for raising money knew no bounds when it came to showing faith in Sheltering Arms Hospital.

At a joint meeting of the Board of Managers and Board of Directors on a hot afternoon in late May of 1979, the vote was unanimous to change Sheltering Arms from an acute care hospital to a rehabilitative care facility. Anxious as the times were in offering a new service at Sheltering Arms, the change was made in a real spirit of cooperation between the women's Board of Managers and the men's Board of Directors. In May of 1980 the merger of members from these two boards into a single Board of Directors permitted a richness in governance. At that juncture, the Board of Managers relinquished its responsibility for day-to-day management of the Hospital and became the Women's Council, with continued responsibility for fund raising, public relations, staff appreciation, and other important functions.

As president of the governing board, Arthur M. Hungerford, Jr., oversaw the conversion; Gilbert Rosenthal served as chairman of building; Dixon Christian was chairman of architectural adaptations for rehab patients; Julia Gray Michaux coordinated the interior decor; Randolph W. McElroy was chairman of contractual arrangements with Richmond Memorial; C. Cotesworth Pinckney's counsel guided the legal process; Isabel Souder's responsibility was to be certain that typical Sheltering Arms patients would be appropriately treated in cooperating sister hospitals; Sarah Keller's committee reviewed requests for financial assistance for rehab patients; Johnnie Lou Terry's responsibility was in public relations; Margaret McElroy was charged to develop a governing structure and to nominate a new board; and Anne Lower and William Reed were chairmen of recruitment. Throughout the transition period, when operating funds were not needed, the board's capable treasurer, John

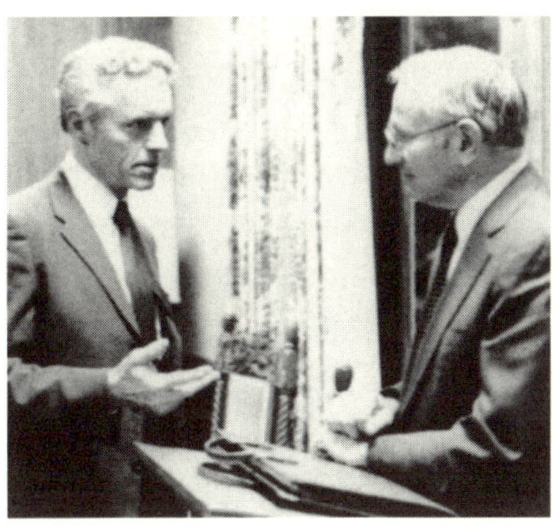

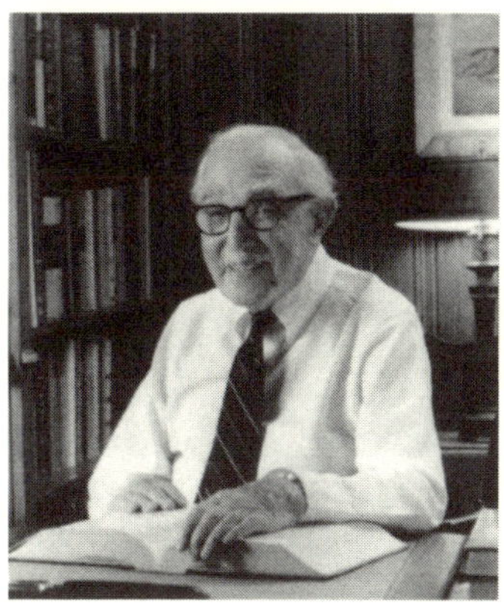

Left: Frederic S. Bocock discusses Hospital finances with Gilbert M. Rosenthal.

Right: Dr. Charles M. Caravati provides a bridge to the medical community.

D. Whitehurst, in conjunction with a vigilant Investment Committee, deposited the endowment income in a "reserve fund."

In 1980 the board elected to use its accumulated endowment to underwrite the conversion of the Hospital for $6,500,000, and did not need to go to the community for capital funds. This was done in the belief that the gifts entrusted to the Hospital through the years had been carefully managed and multiplied for the benefit of the community.

Gordon F. Rainey, Jr., the new board president, coordinated the management with Donald M. Ambrose, the Hospital's part-time administrator from Richmond Memorial, and later with Charles W. Byrd, Jr. Although constant efforts were made to pre-determine cost reimbursement from Blue Cross and other health insurance companies, the board really had made a leap of faith. In changing to rehabilitation medicine, reimbursement for this expensive service was indeed uncertain.

Other board members were involved with the education of staff, volunteers, and support groups into the world of physical rehabilitation. Dr. Charles M. Caravati played a crucial role: to keep the medical community apprised of Sheltering Arms' progress in the transition period, and to help define the need for rehabilitation in the Richmond area.

It was with a certain nostalgia that in May 1980 the doors closed on acute care, a service that Sheltering Arms had been providing so valiantly for nearly a century. Yet there was also a spirit of anticipation and excitement as the Hospital set about remodeling its building and retraining its professional staff for rehabilitation.

Dr. Charles H. Bonner was thirty-three years old in 1980 when the board selected him as the first executive director of Sheltering Arms Rehabilitation Hospital. After completing his residency in physical medicine and rehabilitation, he had remained on the teaching staff at Ohio State University, a leading training program under the chairmanship of Dr. Ernest W. Johnson. During Dr. Bonner's tenure at Sheltering Arms the inpatient census increased and outpatient services were added.

With the shift in care at Sheltering Arms, some of the nurses selected training in rehabilitation, and others went elsewhere to continue in acute care service. Mrs. Virginia King

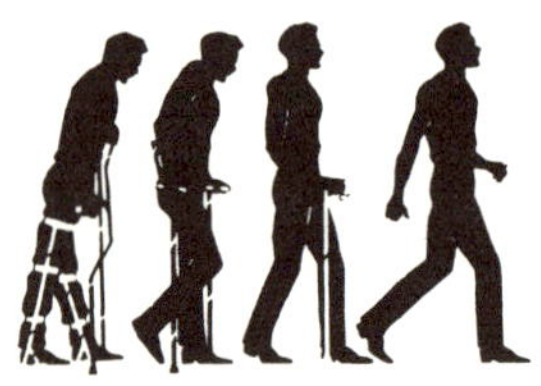

First logo used after the conversion to rehabilitation.

Right: Dr. Charles H. Bonner, first medical director, discusses a coordinated program for a patient with Dr. Robert Mayo, first director of speech pathology.

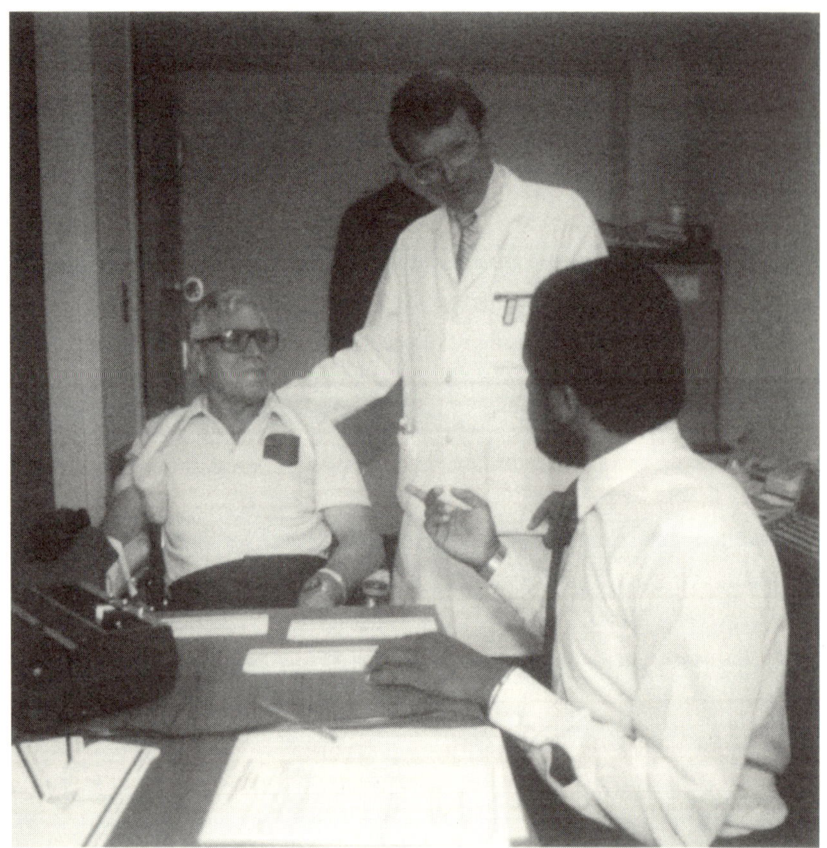

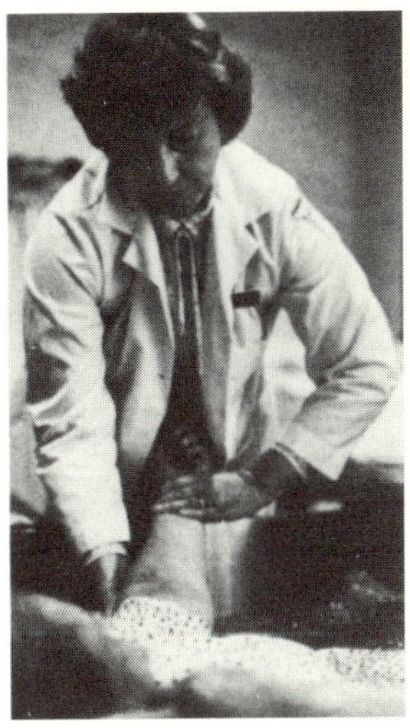

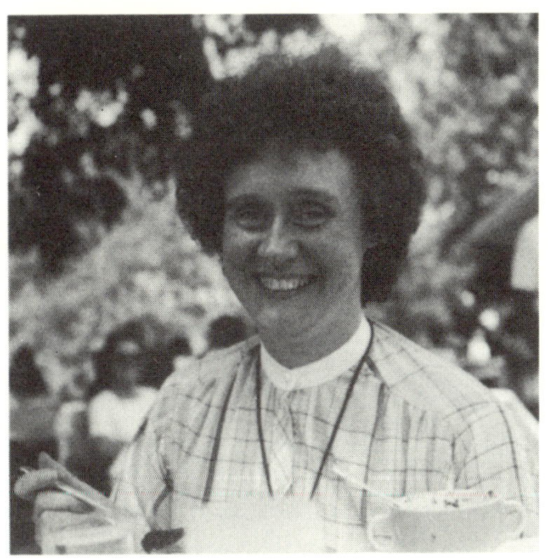

Ann Stitzer (left), the Hospital's first director of physical therapy, and Nancy Dawe (right), the first director of occupational therapy, were key people in the conversion of Sheltering Arms from acute care to rehabilitation.

served as acting head nurse during the transition, and later returned to church work in Africa.

Linda Diehl came from the Medical College of Virginia as director of nursing, and Marjorie Harrison became director of nursing education. Under their guidance, Sheltering Arms instituted "primary care" nursing for its patients.

Other members of the rehab team were four who transferred from Richmond Memorial: Ann Stitzer, director of physical therapy; Anne Bullen, assistant director; Nancy Dawe, director of occupational therapy; Valerie Young, assistant director. Also, Bev Murphey, director of therapeutic recreation; and Becky Mahler, director of social work services.

On a cold Sunday afternoon, January 4, 1981, another dedication ceremony was held at Sheltering Arms Hospital, this time led by Dr. Albert Winn of Second Presbyterian Church. Choristers from St. James's Episcopal Church set the note of gratitude and expectation as many friends of Sheltering Arms gathered for the beginning of its new life. In spite of the winter's chill outside, the Hospital's warmth and color inside welcomed many guests to enjoy tours of the new facility, in which nursing stations and the different therapies were positioned close enough for easy conferences. In addition to an open area for physical therapy and occupational therapy, another interesting feature was the simulated "apartment", where patients could test their skills in independent living with family members before being discharged to return home.

The first patient was admitted the next day, and since then, more than 10,000 people have been given inpatient and outpatient rehabilitation, with the continuing philosophy, "it's the care that counts."

At Sheltering Arms the vision of rehabilitation is to restore each individual to the highest possible level of productivity in order to lead a more independent life. Admittedly, this might not be the same life as before injury or illness, but certainly a life adapted to the new circumstances. Physical, mental, spiritual well-being; recreational pursuits; vocational capacity; family and community reintegration; even volunteer activity, are part of the "continuum of care" fostered by Sheltering Arms.

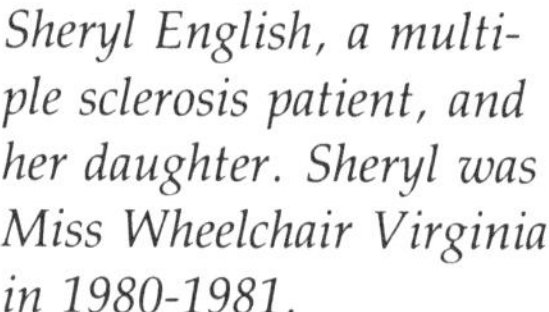

Sheryl English, a multiple sclerosis patient, and her daughter. Sheryl was Miss Wheelchair Virginia in 1980-1981.

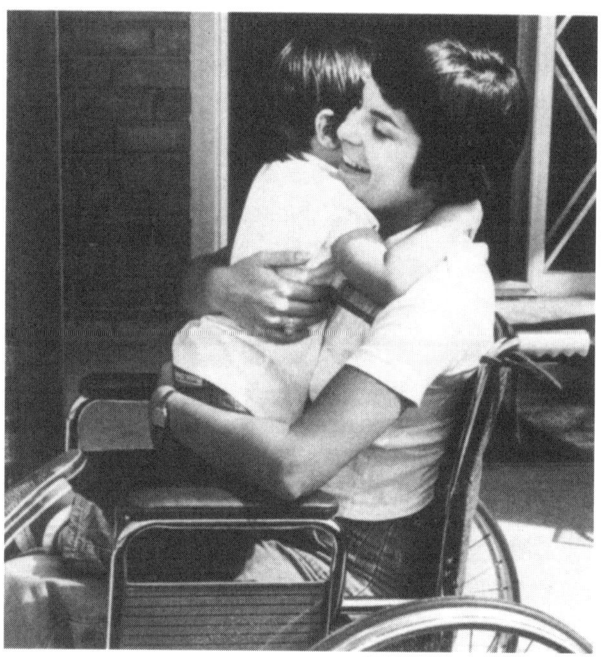

5

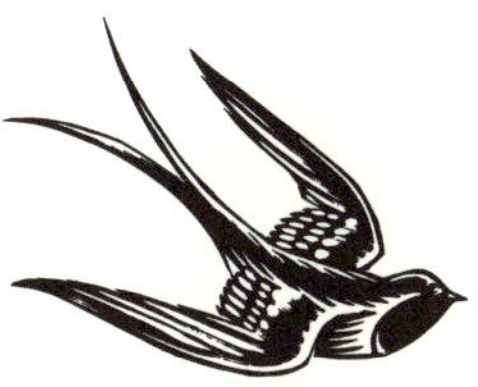

Rehabilitation Success: Building a Future from the Past (1981-1989)

SHELTERING ARMS WAS NOW OFFERING a kind of service unique to Virginia in its comprehensiveness, a service available to all who could benefit, without regard to financial standing or insurance coverage. With all its changes, the Hospital's mission had remained the same: to help people in need of medical care, regardless of their ability to pay.The criteria for inpatient admission were that the patient's condition could be improved by treatment at Sheltering Arms as an inpatient, and that the patient would require treatment by two or more therapies. Those who needed only one therapy would be served as outpatients. And, out of deference to Children's Hospital, Sheltering Arms did not accept patients under eighteen years of age unless Children's Hospital referred them.

This approach to rehabilitation emphasized a coordinated effort by an interdisciplinary team of professionals, all working together in the same place at the same time. The medical doctor was leader of the team and the central player was the patient. Other team members were the rehabilitation nurse, the physical therapist, the occupational therapist, the recreational therapist, the speech pathologist, the psychologist, the dietitian, the pharmacist, the social worker, and the chaplain.

Because rehabilitation treats the whole patient, the family is also included in the rehabilitation process. The importance of educating the family to the problems and expectations of the disabled member is a key to success. Treatment includes finding ways, through therapeutic recreation and vocational services, to aid the patient in reintegration into the community. For a person with a stroke or a spinal cord injury who has been removed from daily life, even the return to home and family can be traumatic. At Sheltering Arms, therefore, a goal of reintegration is established early in the treatment plan.

In 1983 alone, 194 people were admitted to Sheltering Arms for an average stay of forty days. In its first two years, the Hospital had served an average of more than twenty-two patients a day, for an occupancy rate of almost ninety-one percent. The patients' average age was fifty-eight, and nearly seventy-five percent of them came from the greater Richmond area. Thirty-seven percent had private insurance and fifty-seven percent of these patients had coverage under either Medicare or Medicaid; yet $435,000 was given in financial assistance for the many areas that were not reimbursable. The largest single diagnosis for the patients, fifty-six percent, was CVA or stroke. Other diagnoses, in order of decreasing frequency, were spinal cord injury, traumatic brain injury, other neurological problems, amputation, arthritis, and orthopedic problems.

The Board of Directors was gratified by the ever-increasing number of patients and the steady support of public donations, but as laymen they also felt Sheltering Arms should

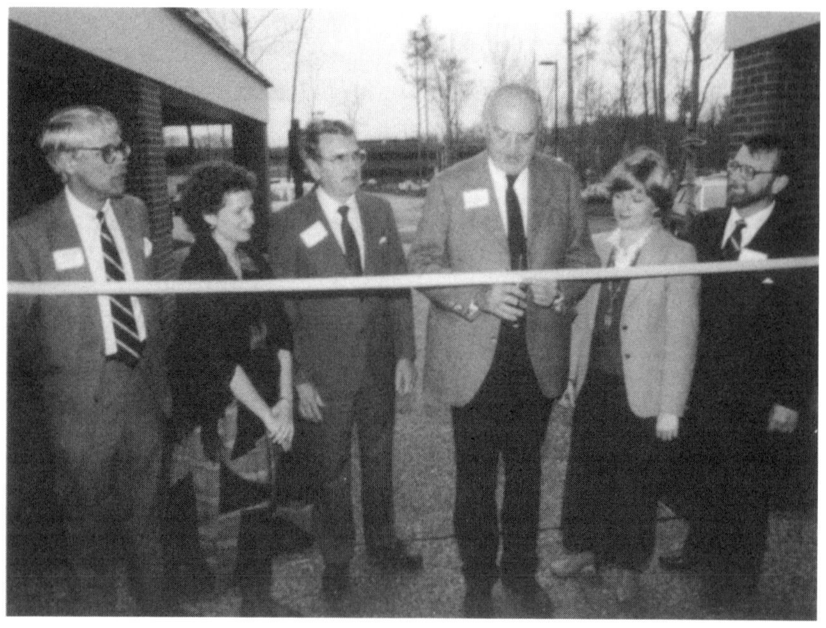

James C. Wheat, Jr., cuts the ribbon at opening of Stony Point outpatient facility. Looking on, from left: C. Cotesworth Pinckney, Ana Mieres, Richard C. Craven, Jane Brooke, Dr. Henry H. Stonnington.

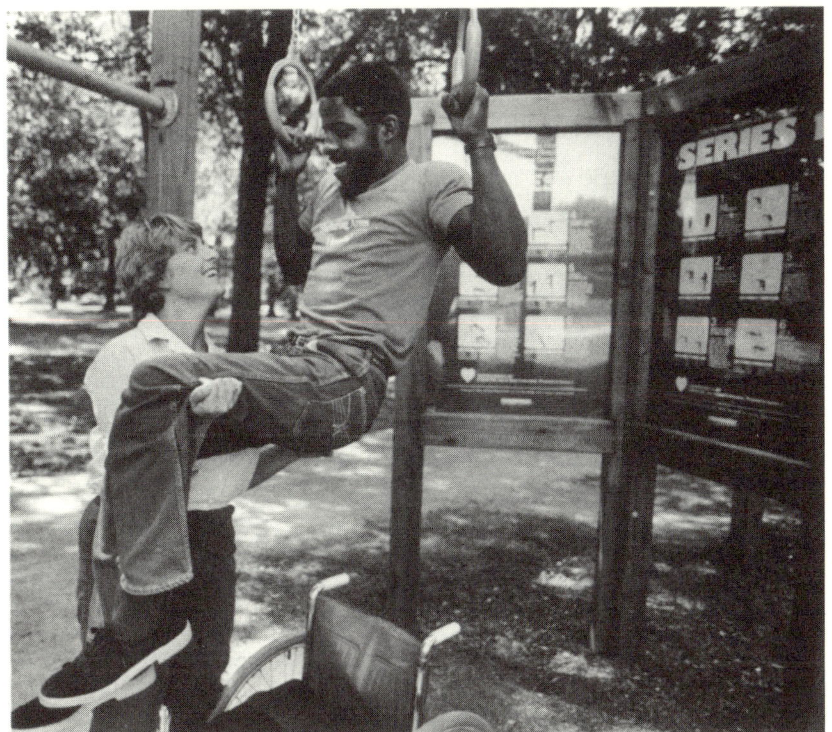

Doris Dickerson, TR, and Charlie Snead, patient, at exercise trail for disabled and able-bodied citizens.

be managed by a full-time professional administrator. In September 1982 they selected for the post Richard C. Craven, who had been associate director of the Sister Kenny Institute in Minneapolis. Mr. Craven's unflappable nature, warm-heartedness, and personnel skills were exceedingly valuable in building a new organization for Sheltering Arms. In the later 1980s his capable leadership resolved many of the stresses caused by the rapid growth of the Hospital's staff and the prolonged construction of the building expansion.

As the decade continued, Sheltering Arms re-established its own Medical Records Department, which had been shared with Richmond Memorial since 1965. In 1984 an audiology service was added, and a head injury program was initiated. Through a cooperative effort with Union Theological Seminary and Richmond Memorial, Sheltering Arms also set up an exercise trail for both able-bodied and disabled citizens in a park on Westwood Avenue. And to enhance the patients' stay in the hospital, a project to exhibit works of art (often donated by the artist) was organized by Nancy Thalhimer, then president of the Women's Council.

As the number of outpatients grew, the yearly inpatient occupancy remained at more than ninety percent, and there was always a waiting list. Everyone became increasingly aware of the need for additional space. It was time to review phase two of the 1977 master site plan, and to consider either expansion on the Palmyra site or building elsewhere. Sheltering Arms approached other non-profit hospitals to consider available locations; in the end, the board voted to stay at Palmyra, to increase the number of inpatient beds to 40, and to add space for other programs, including a therapeutic pool. The latter would be open to the disabled community in Richmond, as well as to Sheltering Arms patients. The entire project would be paid for by income reserves from the endowment.

The Sheltering Arms logo since 1985.

Right: New therapeutic pool for the disabled opened in 1988, offering special programs for both inpatients and outpatients. Robert White, spinal cord injured, and Emma Dial, arthritic, work with therapists.

Under the leadership of Dixon Christian, plans were carefully laid for the expansion, and a mission statement was developed to reaffirm goals and to establish priorities for expanding programs at Sheltering Arms.

As word of Sheltering Arms' successful treatment of patients spread, an increased number of volunteers gave time and talent to this special institution. Two hundred of these loyal supporters spent more than a thousand hours a month helping in many ways other than fund raising: answering the telephone, escorting patients, and working in the various therapy areas.

Since 1889, a high point of each year at Sheltering Arms has been Donation Day. Early in November friends of the Hospital gather to bring the fruits of their fund raising efforts, to share the ongoing saga of Sheltering Arms, and to be renewed themselves by the many examples of triumph of the human spirit.

In the fifty years since the founding of her King's Daughters Circle in 1931, Mrs. Roy Caudle's methods of inviting donations to Sheltering Arms had become legendary. Give a person a lift in your car, she said, and mention the kitty for Sheltering Arms on the dash. Much in the tradition of Mrs.

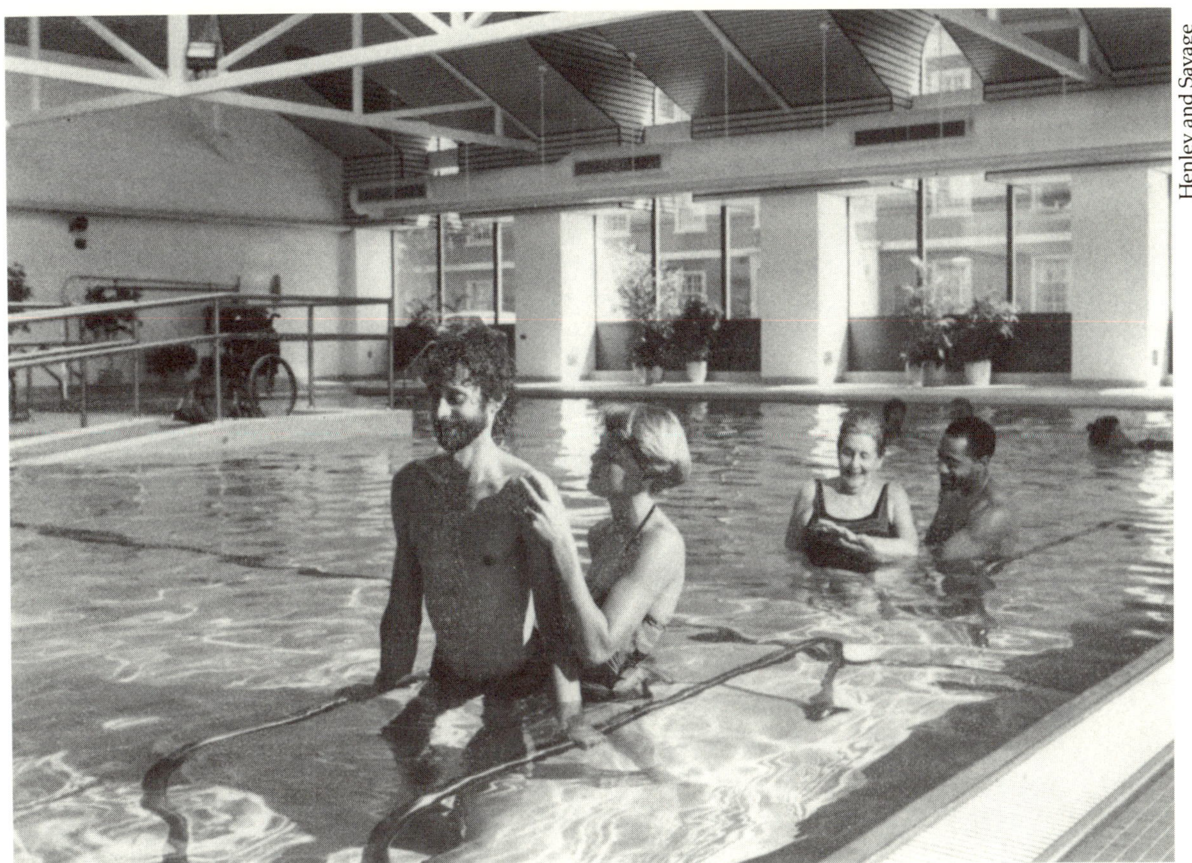

Henley and Savage

George T. King, Mrs. Caudle had no qualms about telephoning several dozen businessmen on the Southside to remind them that it was donation season for Sheltering Arms. These were "Mrs. Caudle's men," not to be solicited by anyone else.

Who of Mrs. Caudle's Hope Circle and invited guests could ever forget the temperance-minded Christmas parties at the Old Stone House in Forest Hill Park and the place to slip folded dollar bills into a model hospital "cot"?

Annually, countless individuals, church and community groups, and businesses large and small express their appreciation for the work of Sheltering Arms Hospital. It is through their gifts of money and service that over $800,000 worth of free care was given to needy patients this year by the Financial Assistance Committee.

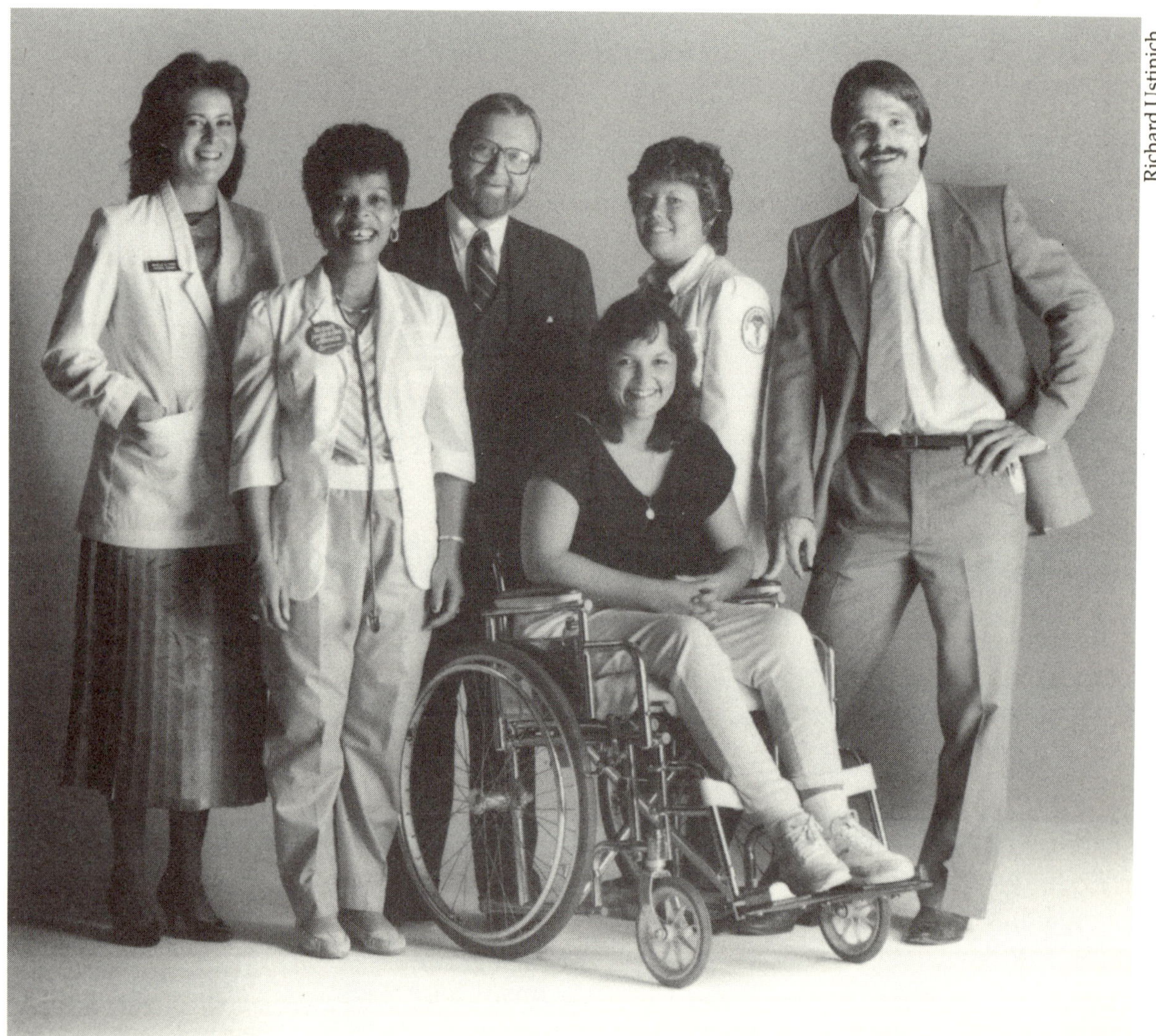

Richard Ustinich

As the number of patients increased, Sheltering Arms added another physician to the active medical staff. Henry H. Stonnington joined Sheltering Arms on a part-time basis in 1985 as the first medical director of the new day rehab program. Austrian by birth, Dr. Stonnington received his training in physical medicine and rehabilitation at the Mayo Clinic in Rochester, Minnesota, where he was an associate professor from 1979 to 1983. He also served at the Medical College of Virginia as chairman of the Department of Rehabilitation Medicine from 1983 to 1988. In 1986 he became the second medical director of Sheltering Arms Rehabilitation Hospital.

The outpatient service, which had grown tremendously under Dr. Herbert W. Park (1987 through 1988), now demanded the increase in Sheltering Arms' active medical staff to four doctors. Dr. Stonnington attracted Drs. Albert M. Jones, Manmohan Khokhar, and Jane Pendleton Wootton to join Sheltering Arms' full-time staff after completion of their residency training at the Medical College of Virginia (1988 and 1989). This full-time staff is augmented by seventy consulting physicians.

To fulfill its mission of offering a continuum of rehabilitation services, Sheltering Arms opened a Day Rehabilitation Program at Stony Point in February 1986. James C. Wheat, Jr., Virginia Commissioner for the Rights of the Disabled, was the keynote speaker at the dedication. This satellite facility at Stony Point, south of the James River, incorporated a full day of therapy, lunch, rest space, and transportation for patients who, having been discharged from a hospital, needed intensive care but not 24-hour nursing care. In 1989 the Day Rehabilitation

Far left: Deborah Fossé, at center, with part of her rehab team: Michelle Favero, PT; Jean Hicks, RN; Dr. Henry H. Stonnington, medical director; Carolyn Costello, OT; and Dr. Michael Martelli, psychology.

Lower: Sheltering Arms' full-time staff physicians, trained in rehabilitation medicine: Dr. Albert Jones, Dr. Jane Wootton, Dr. Manmohan Khokhar.

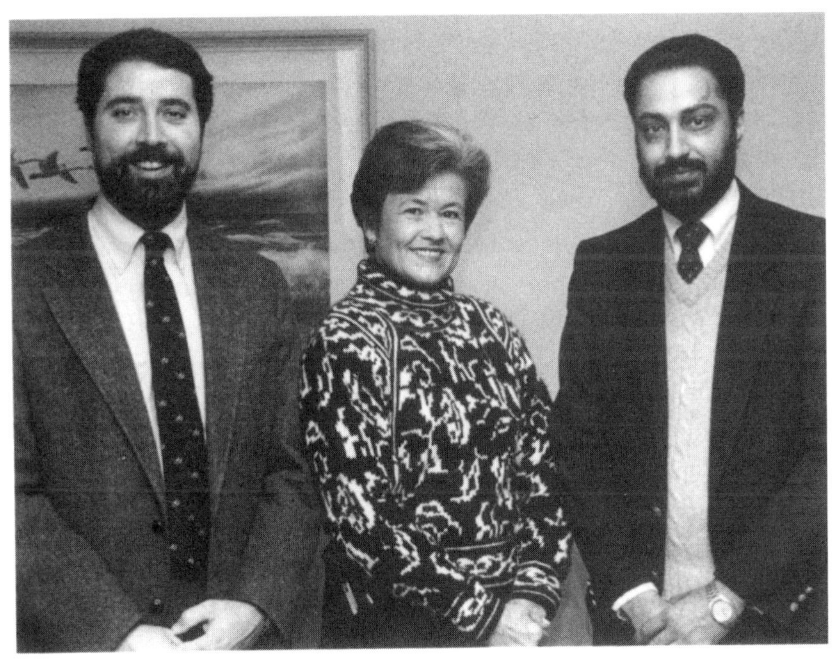

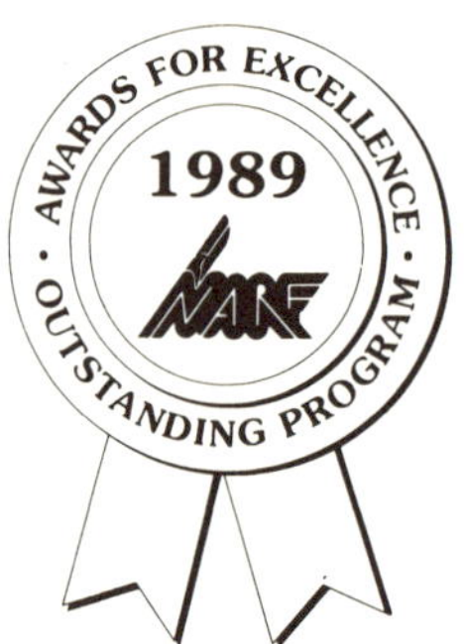

The Day Rehabilitation Program received national recognition in 1989.

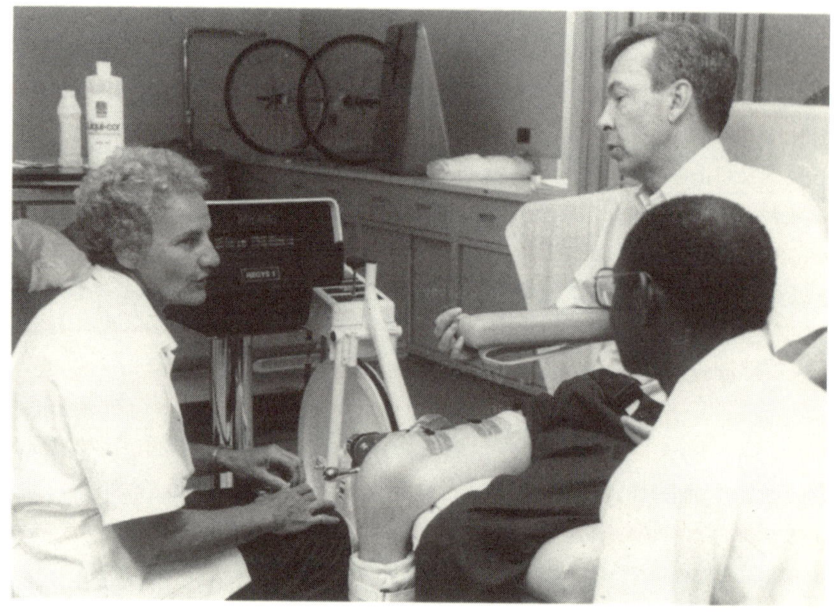

Right: The Florence Nightingale Circle gave the State's first Regys I functional electrical stimulator to the Hospital in 1988. Here being used by Dixon Christian, in consultation with physical therapists Anne Bullen and James Bell.

Program received national recognition by the National Association of Rehabilitation Facilities (NARF) as the outstanding medical rehabilitation program. Sheltering Arms was honored for providing "dynamic, innovative rehabilitation for community reentry through the integration of patients' lives in the community and the restorative rehabilitation process."

Also located at Stony Point is the Vocational Industrial Services department of Sheltering Arms. For those patients who have suffered a job-related accident, the Vocational Industrial Services offers evaluation and a comprehensive daily routine of "work hardening," job adaptation, and employment counseling. At this end of the continuum a disabled person can also regain personal self-esteem, enhancing life while motivating vocational independence.

To manage the many outpatient activities in two areas, ten miles apart, Sheltering Arms added an associate administrator. Michael McDonnell came from rehabilitation facilities in eastern Pennsylvania to take charge of Sheltering Arms' outpatient services in 1986. Mr. McDonnell has been largely responsible for the growth and efficient operation of Sheltering Arms' Day

Rehabilitation Program and Vocational Industrial Services at Stony Point.

Back at 1311 Palmyra, for two long years, the Hospital underwent further expansion of its programs and its facility. Completion was celebrated triumphantly with a Grand Opening on September 18, 1988. The new east wing of Sheltering Arms was dedicated with an invocation by Dr. Jack D. Spiro of Congregation Beth Ahabah; commendations by Mayor Geline B. Williams from the City of Richmond; and remarks by Jeanne P. Baliles, wife of the Governor, who spoke on the contribution of disabled citizens to the life of our community.

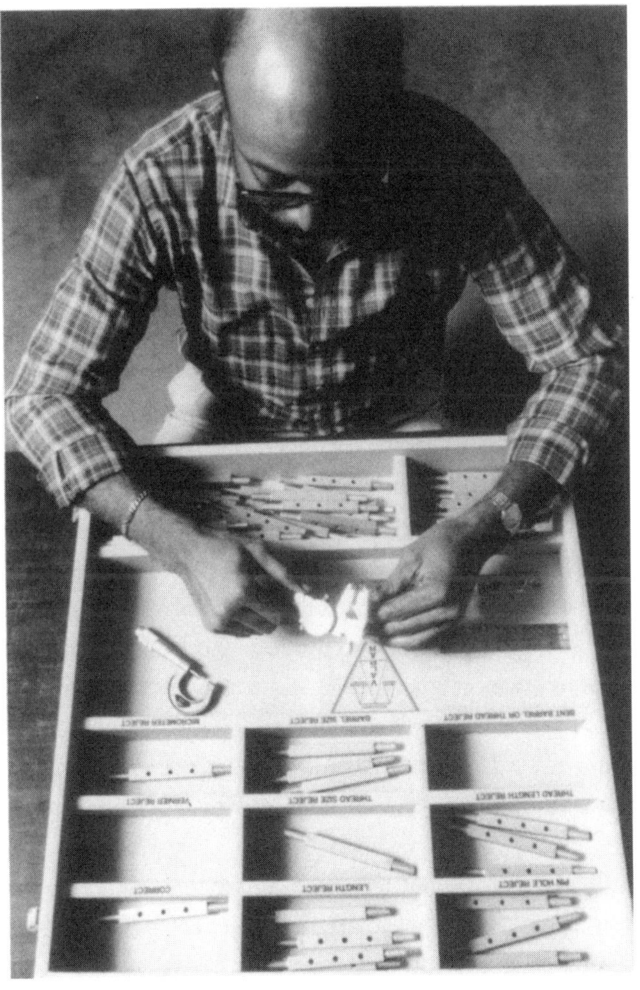

Johnny Raspberry, a City fireman, undergoes rehabilitation at Vocational Industrial Services.

Since its beginning as a rehabilitation facility in January 1981, more than 10,000 individuals have received either inpatient or outpatient service at Sheltering Arms. More than one-third of them were treated between October 1987 and September 1989. In the labor-intensive field of rehabilitation, the full-time staff has grown to almost 190, eighty-five percent of whom are highly trained professionals.

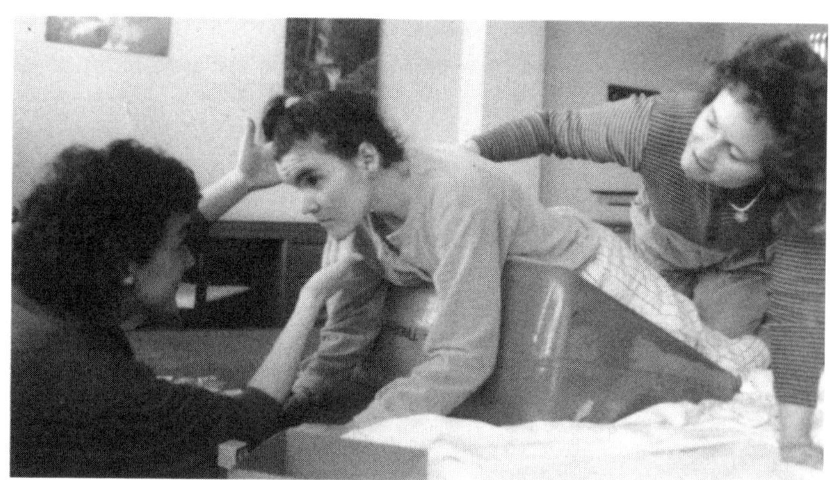

Edie Robinson receives therapy from brain injury team therapists, Anne Lacy, OT, and Sarah Bates, PT.

In this period of growth in staff and programs, the Hospital enjoyed the quiet guidance of Jean Dickinson, a clinical psychologist, as president of the Board of Directors. Mrs. Dickinson was as enthusiastic in recognizing and supporting the staff as she was vigilant in the board's responsibility for professional accreditation and the assurance of quality of care.

By the mid-eighties professional responsibility for the quality of hospital care was formalized in departments of Quality Assurance. This was both an administrative function and a responsibility of boards of trustees. Sheltering Arms was fortunate to have Dr. Edwin Lawrence Kendig, Jr., an eminent Richmond physician, to guide and advise the board and administration.

Public awareness of the needs of the disabled community has significantly increased from a scant decade ago when organizations like Sheltering Arms first advocated barrier-free environments. In 1987, Mayor Roy A. West proclaimed National Rehabilitation Week in Richmond and named Sheltering Arms as its local sponsor. In this role as advocate to represent the needs of the disabled, Sheltering Arms formed a citizens' Consumer Advisory Council in early 1989, with several former patients as members.

The Sheltering Arms goal to help people return to the workplace despite their disabilities can be augmented by an accessible independent living arrangement. Sheltering Arms is committed to a "continuum of care" for patients with disabilities, and transitional living is one end of the continuum. Sheltering Arms is studying transitional living as a further way to help its patients regain productive roles in the community.

In working toward its goal of restoring patients to a full life, Sheltering Arms knows that a person's "wellness" involves the spirit, as well as the mind and body. Therefore, with its continued faith in a higher power, the Hospital hopes to establish its own interfaith chapel and chaplaincy service for patients and their families, staff and volunteers.

Dr. Henry Betts, medical director of the Rehabilitation Institute of Chicago, had served as a consultant to Sheltering Arms in the 1970s. He returned to Sheltering Arms for the Founders Day centennial celebration on February 9, 1989, and made the following affirmation:

> *"It was very thrilling for me to see Sheltering Arms again, and to observe the wonderful progress which has been made here. All of you have done a remarkable thing by creating an enterprise which will reach out to help thousands of people in the future. The dedication of your board and your staff is perfectly evident. It radiates through the events you have and from the people one meets here."*

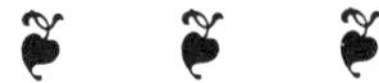

Epilogue

It has been noted that as organizational entities, many hospitals are moving away from their historic roots of charity. The healing mission is at times being replaced with a business ethic.

Perhaps Sheltering Arms is an exception to this trend. It still offers quality care regardless of patients' ability to pay. Together with like-minded institutions, it still emphasizes the dignity of the individual; it still enjoys the enthusiasm of valued staff and volunteers; and its philosophy still includes the spiritual element. The key to its survival and its growth may be that Sheltering Arms is both flexible and vigilant. Sheltering Arms adheres to a mission that adapts to the needs of humanity.

At the benchmark of 100 years, the story of Sheltering Arms endures as a story of caring. It is the story of a hospital led by an inspiring founder and built by the vision and support of private citizens throughout the decades—all dedicated to caring for one's fellow human beings. The result has been healing of mind, body and spirit by virtue of the care given here by hundreds of dedicated professionals, volunteers, and friends.

In Sheltering Arms' centennial year, the human spirit continues to triumph at this hospital with a heart.

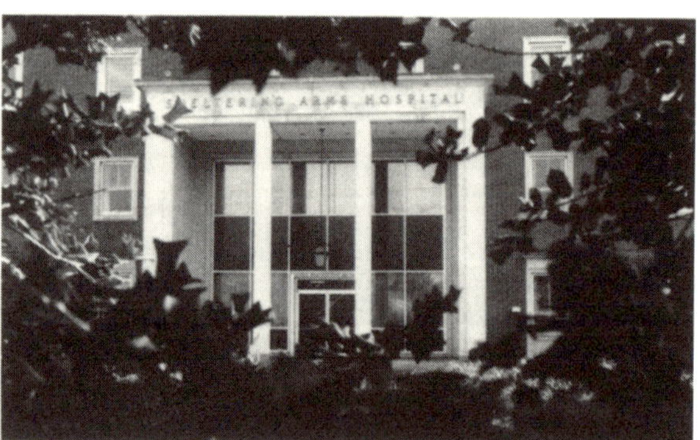

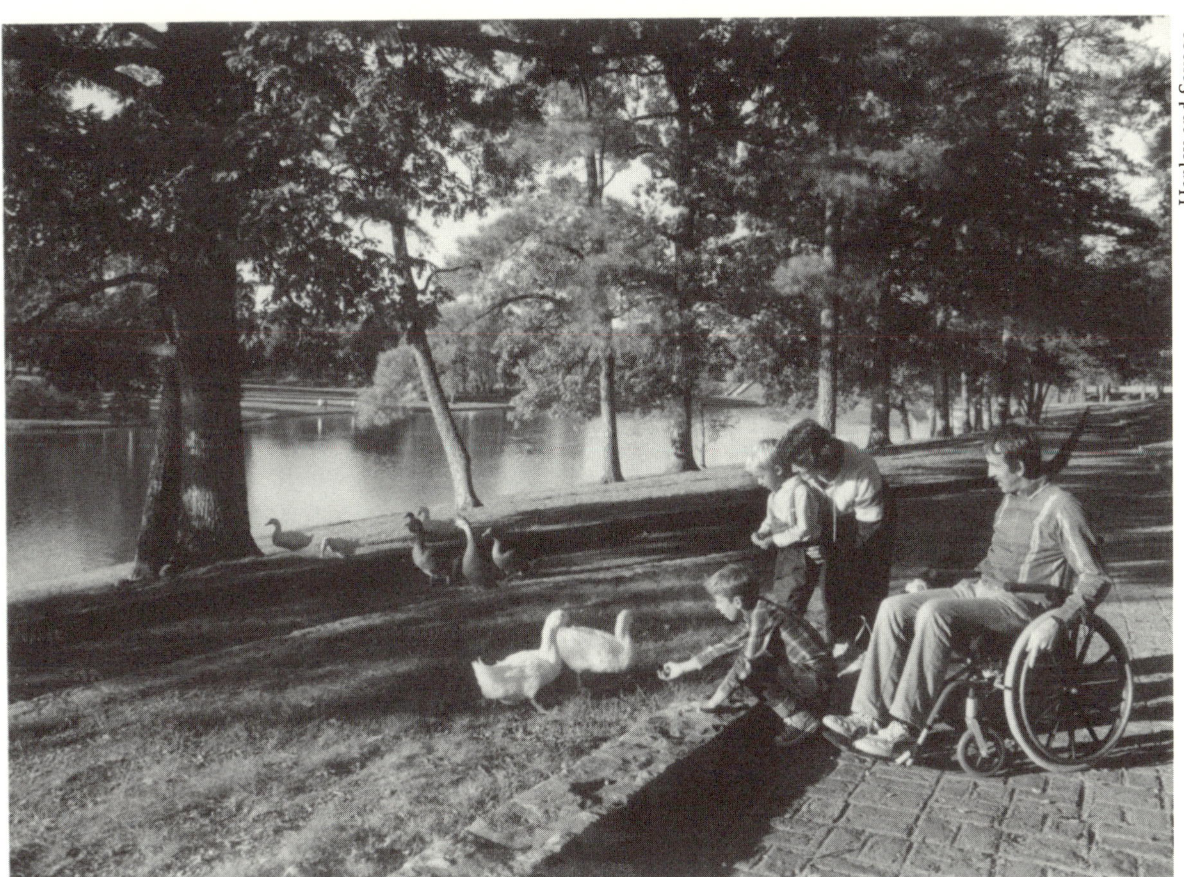

Henley and Savage

The Pletcher family exemplifies how rehabilitation can help people who survive severe accidents and multiple injuries. Chip, the father, experienced brain injury, was rehabilitated and returned to his work as a computer design engineer.

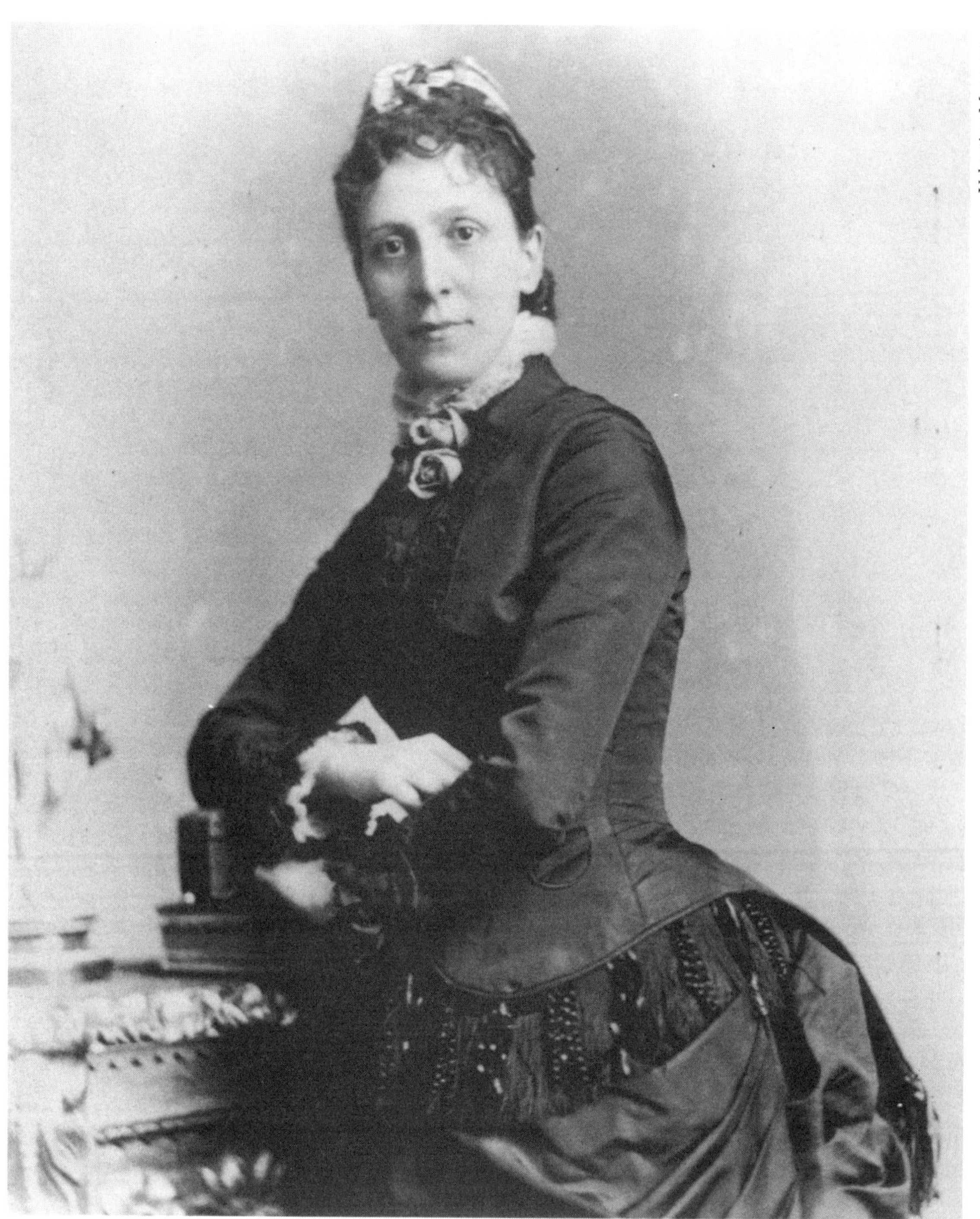

Valentine Museum

Rebekah Dulaney Peterkin

6

Biographical Vignettes

THE PETERKIN FAMILY

WHO WAS THIS LIVELY WOMAN who died of unknown cause near Baltimore, the city of her father's family? "The world is better for the life of Miss Rebekah Peterkin. There can be no grander tribute than this, there could be no surer claim to blissful immortality," said the obituary in the Richmond Dispatch. It went on to say, "few lives indeed have ever been more earnestly. . . devoted to ministrations of good than that which has just been ended (July 26, 1891). The greatest pleasures of her life found origin in the joy and comfort she brought to others."

Rebekah was the youngest child of the Reverend Joshua Peterkin, D.D. (1814-1892) and Elizabeth Howard Hanson (1820-1910). She was born in Berryville, Virginia, on September 24, 1849. Her only brother, George William Peterkin, was born in Clear Spring, Washington County, Maryland, on March 21, 1841, and died in 1916. An older sister did not live beyond adolescence.

Mary Wingfield Scott describes Dr. Peterkin as one of the most beloved clergymen who ever lived in Richmond. From 1855 until his death in 1892 he was rector of St. James's Episcopal Church, then at Fifth and Marshall Streets. From 1860 to 1910 the Peterkins' simple and unpretentious home was at 705 East Leigh Street, just five blocks from the church in which Rebekah's sewing circle met to plan the founding of Sheltering Arms Hospital.

A missionary spirit guided the whole Peterkin family. Dr. Peterkin had been instrumental in establishing St. Mark's, Grace

Church, and St. Philip's, sending members from his own congregation to strengthen new parishes further west in the city. Dr. Peterkin was personally diligent in attending the sick and quarantined of his flock. Rebekah no doubt felt the grateful response to his ministrations; she identified the suffering in her father's parish and determined to do something to relieve it. At that time Richmond's "downtown" included a relatively small area, those sections annexed by the city toward the end of the eighteenth century. We might presume that the parish was bordered on the south by the James River, on the west by Lombardy Street, on the north by Hospital Street and the cemetery, and on the east by Shockoe Valley.

Rebekah's brother George had served in the Confederate Army in Stonewall Jackson's second division, and on General Lee's staff. After the war, finding business not to his liking, he chose to attend seminary and to devote his life to the church. George was consecrated as the first bishop of the Diocese of West Virginia in 1878, shortly after the death of his young wife,

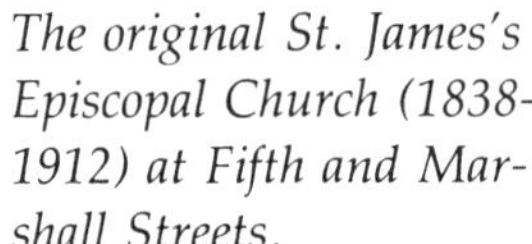

The original St. James's Episcopal Church (1838-1912) at Fifth and Marshall Streets.

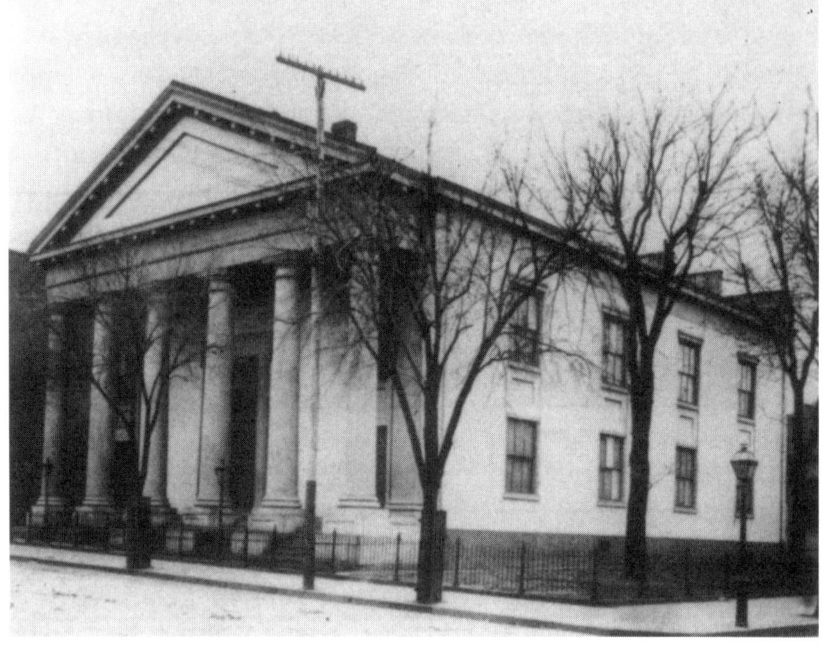

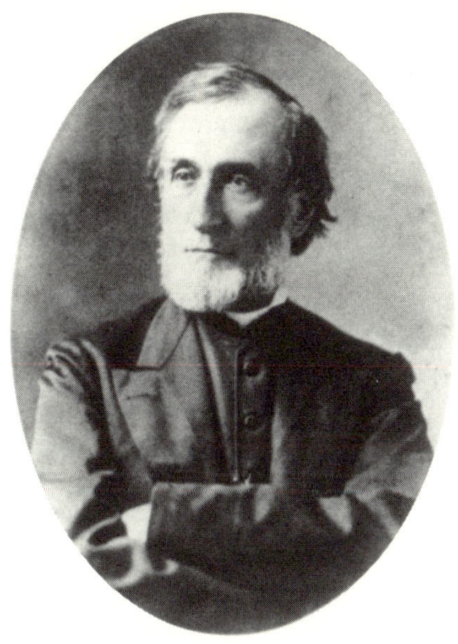
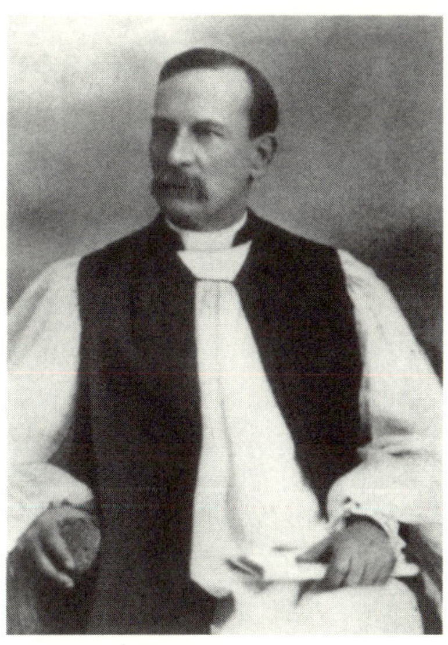

Left: The Reverend Dr. Joshua Peterkin.

Right: The Right Reverend George Peterkin.

Constance Gardner Lee. He lived the rest of his life in Parkersburg, West Virginia, but in 1884 he married Marion McIntosh Stewart, daughter of John Stewart of "Brook Hill," Henrico County, Virginia.

Bishop Peterkin has been described as an able administrator and one whose endless energy was well suited to tackle the many problems of the undeveloped state and Diocese of West Virginia. He realized that medical and surgical care should be made available at moderate cost to coal miners from isolated areas. To answer the need for a hospital, Bishop Peterkin selected the railroad area of Hansford, twenty miles up the river from Charleston, to build a free hospital in 1887. He called it "The Sheltering Arms," and it continued operations there until 1924.

Rebekah's mother was also dedicated to the care of the sick and the indigent. She had been a volunteer nurse at Capt. Sally Tompkins' C.S.A. hospital during the Civil War, and for many years, Mrs. Peterkin was president of the Protestant Episcopal Church Home, incorporated in 1875 for the benefit of indigent Episcopal ladies. In spite of the grief of losing her daughter Rebekah in one year and her husband the next, Mrs. Peterkin remained faithful to Sheltering Arms Hospital during the 1890s and was president of the executive board from 1900 to 1910.

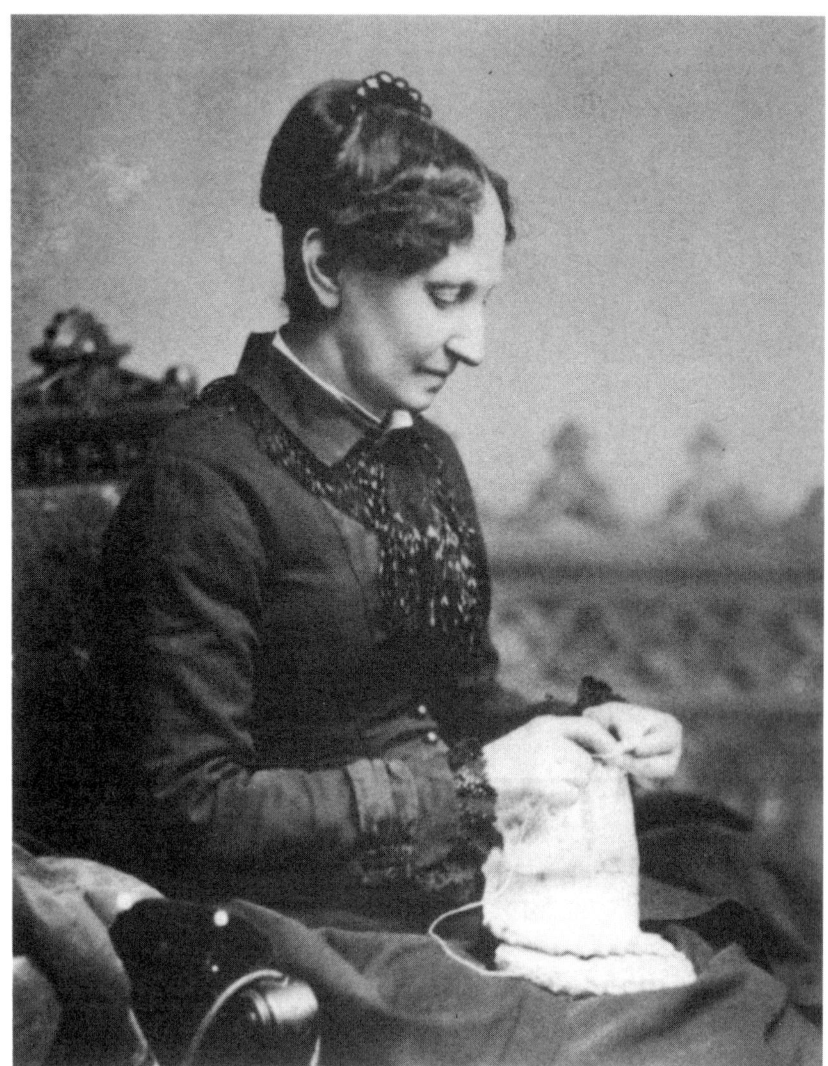

Elizabeth Hanson Peterkin, wife of Joshua and mother of Rebekah and George, ministered to the sick and indigent from the Civil War to 1910.

MOSES DRURY HOGE, JR., M.D. (1861-1920)
First Doctor of Sheltering Arms

As a young man who had just finished medical training in Heidelberg, Germany, in 1886, Dr. Hoge was persuaded to help Miss Peterkin in the management of her newly established free hospital in Richmond. The son of the Reverend Moses D. Hoge, D.D., longtime minister of Second Presbyterian Church in Richmond, the younger Hoge knew well the need for medical care downtown.

As a private physician, Dr. Hoge maintained an office at 305 East Grace Street and was a member of the faculty of the University College of Medicine (now MCV) as Professor of Pathology, Histology, and Urinology, from 1893 to 1901. The author of articles in learned journals, Dr. Hoge was reported in magazines and newspapers for his interest in laboratory methods for identifying tubercle bacilli, examining urinary sediment, studying osteo problems, and the use of the new Roentgen rays (x-rays) to diagnose hand injuries.

When Dr. Hoge married Alice Page Aylett in 1895, the newspaper described him as one of the city's outstanding physicians. He became president of the Richmond Academy of Medicine in 1898, and served at the Office of the Board of Health for many years, always concerned with infectious diseases and the medical inspection of schools. He was also on the Board of Directors of the Children's Home Society of Virginia and served on the Board of Trustees of the Richmond City Schools from 1904 until his death in 1920.

Newspaper headlines of 1906 proclaimed that "Richmond has motor car craze—some 78 cars on the streets." Dr. Hoge's personal life reflected a fascination with automobiles; he served on the executive committee of the new Richmond Automobile Club. Exciting as the new machine was, his records show that he was seeing terrible injuries, even in children, caused by automobiles.

From his student days in Germany, Dr. Hoge developed a lifelong interest in that country and in German activities in Richmond.

We know Dr. Hoge had at least one daughter, a civic leader in this city, Alice Hoge (Mrs. E.D. Waller) and a son, William Aylett Hoge, who lived at the Aylett ancestral home "Mt. Holly" in Virginia. Dr. Hoge's wife of 25 years, Alice Page Aylett, was the great-great granddaughter of Patrick Henry. She died at her home on West Avenue in 1941.

According to the treasurer of Sheltering Arms, Mrs. George T. King, Dr. Hoge made continual donations to the Hospital. In 1902, when the newspaper reported on Donation Day at "the Sheltering Arms Free Hospital," Dr. Hoge's gifts were listed among those of others. Upon his death in 1920, $500 was bequeathed to Sheltering Arms.

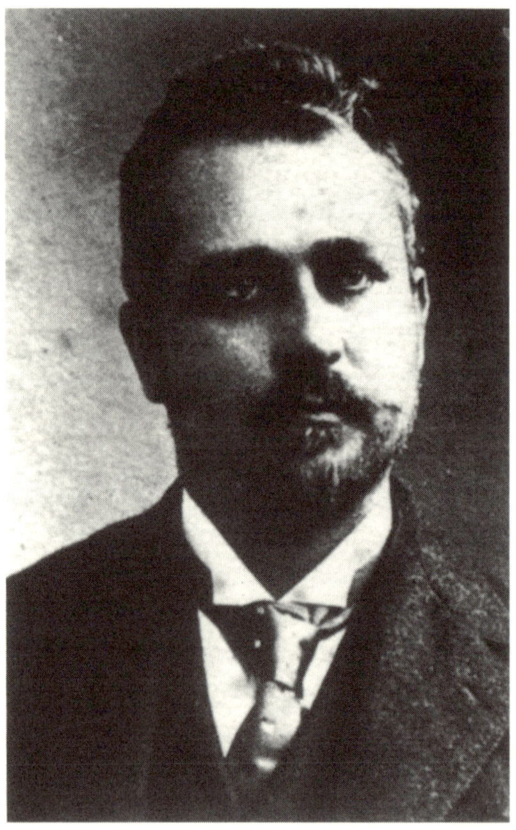

Medical College of Virginia Archives

Dr. Moses D. Hoge, Jr., the first of generations of physicians to donate their services at Sheltering Arms.

FRANCES BRANCH SCOTT (1861-1937)

"Where there is little money, there must be a lot of work: Sheltering Arms Hospital."

AS PRESIDENT OF THE BOARD of Sheltering Arms, Miss Scott addressed the forty-eighth Founders Day program on February 16, 1937; it was the last time this strong leader would appear at a public gathering of any kind. When she died at her home on Palm Sunday, March 21, 1937, she ended twenty-seven years of leadership and almost half a century of devoted work on behalf of Sheltering Arms.

"Miss Boxie," as she was affectionately known, was the daughter of Major Frederic R. Scott, C.S.A., a native of County Donegal, Ireland, and Sarah Frances Branch of Petersburg. The family moved to Richmond in 1872 and soon built the gracious mansion at 712 West Franklin Street, facing Monroe Park. This was to be Miss Boxie's home for the rest of her life, and the center of much social activity and charity work. Her brother, Frederic William Scott, and many nephews, nephews-in-law, and nieces for the next two generations would contribute time, talent, and treasure to Sheltering Arms. Miss Boxie's reign would span the First World War, the influenza epidemic, the 19th Amendment to the Constitution granting women the right to vote, Lindbergh's flight across the Atlantic, the roaring twenties, and the Great Depression. During this time, the lady board of managers would actively manage this great charity hospital, which gave such fine care to thousands of patients.

Miss Boxie was at the Hospital nearly every day, often in consultation with Miss Natalie Curtis, superintendent, and Miss Hazel Hill, assistant superintendent. Miss Boxie and the medical director, Dr. Margaret Nolting, knew personally almost all the doctors who attended patients at Sheltering Arms. Although very generous by nature, Miss Boxie was strictly frugal in the management of Sheltering Arms' funds. And with good reason, for the treasurer, Mrs. George T. King, spent her life raising the

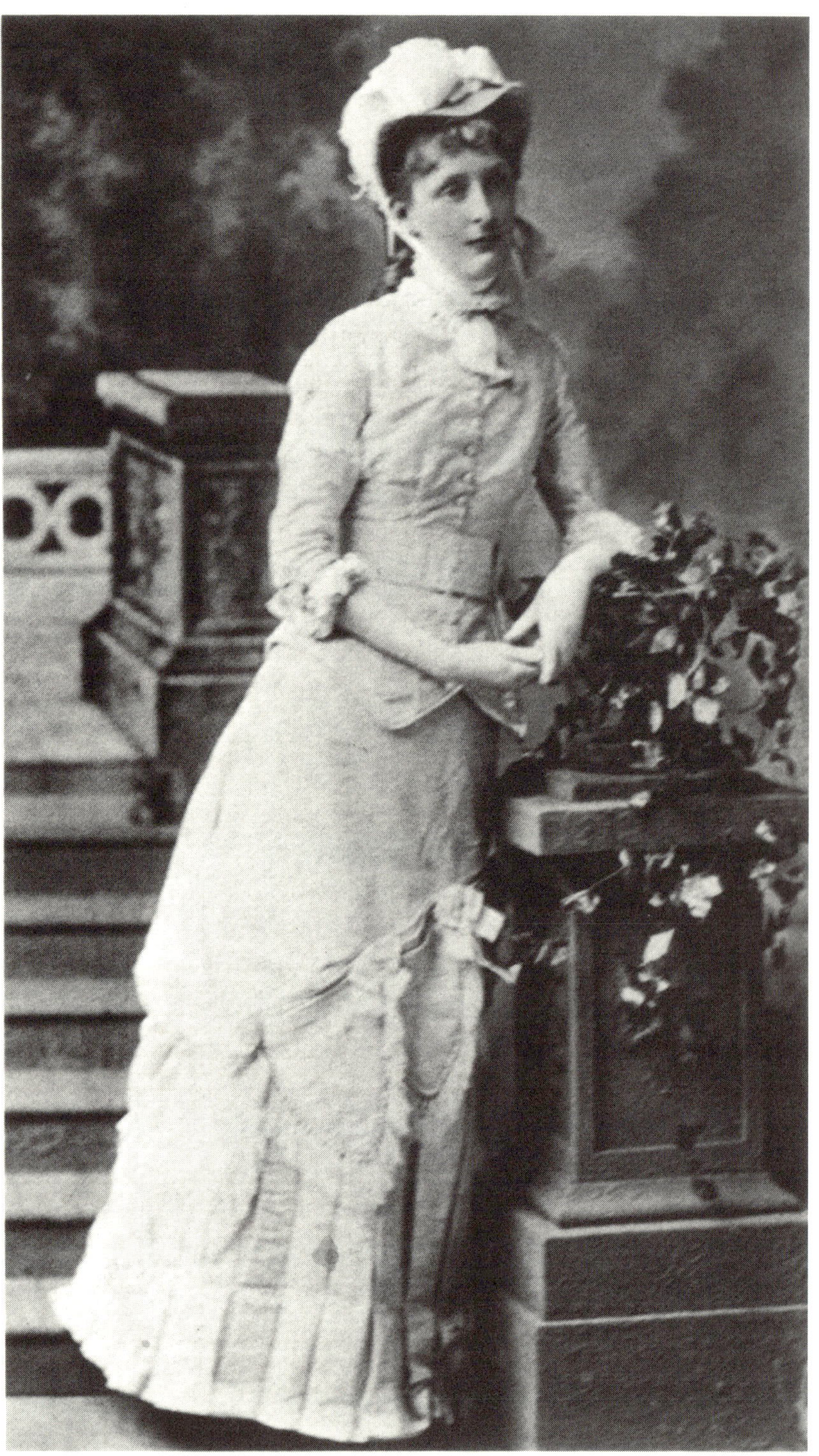

Miss Frances Branch Scott as a young woman, whom Rebekah Peterkin enlisted in 1891 to help lead the new hospital on Fourteenth Street.

funds to pay the Hospital bills, "wringing the hearts of financiers on Main Street." The need to care for the poor was great and the responsibility of these capable women to stretch a dollar was serious business.

According to Miss Boxie's obituary in the Richmond newspaper, *"Rebekah Peterkin first interested Miss Scott in charitable work. At her request, Miss Scott agreed to work with the Financial Committee, which had been set up to raise funds for the hospital. She was a member of the original hospital board. Of the 31 women who were on that hospital board, only one, Mrs. King, was still alive in the spring of 1937."*

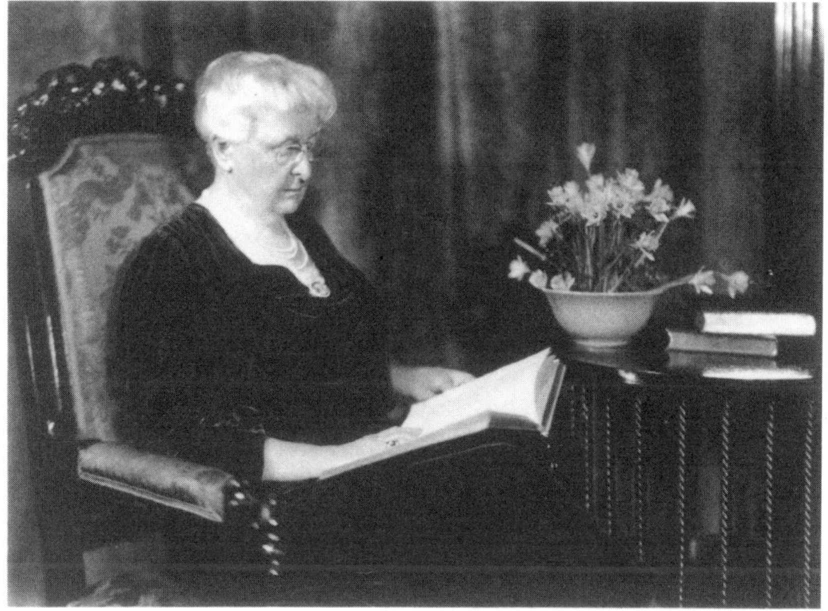

Miss Scott in later years after a lifetime of volunteer service to needy people, including 27 years as president of the Hospital's executive board.

As friends tell of the founding of another needed institution, Pine Camp Sanatorium, they reveal Miss Boxie's concern for the poor and needy. Another obituary confirmed her empathy for the needy: *"In 1908 doctors at Sheltering Arms discovered a fifteen-year-old girl to be tubercular. There were no facilities at the hospital or in Richmond for treating tubercular patients and so Miss Scott offered to pay for her care in a private home. After several months the girl died. In the months during which she lingered between life and death, the girl had won the affection of Miss Scott who resolved that facilities for treating tubercular patients had to be erected in Richmond. She called a meeting of friends in the parlor of her home and there the idea for Pine Camp Sanatorium was born.*" From this movement resulted the Richmond Tuberculosis Association, which supervised the operation of Pine Camp until 1916, when it was taken over by the city.

Miss Scott was also part of the group of Richmonders who established the Fresh Air Camp, maintained in Charles City County by the Alpha Circle of The King's Daughters, of which she was a member.

Frances Branch Scott was beloved by a large circle of relatives and friends who held her in high esteem as a woman of cultivated intellect, of rare distinction in appearance and manner, and whose broad sympathies had led her to devote much of her time to the welfare of the ill and the poor. Through her work, she left an indelible mark on the people and the history of Sheltering Arms Hospital.

❦ ❦ ❦

THE FLORENCE NIGHTINGALE CIRCLE
First Auxiliary, Founded 1910

THE FIRST ORGANIZED SHELTERING ARMS AUXILIARY, The Florence Nightingale Circle, was founded in 1910 when Frances Branch Scott suggested to Miss Josephine Sizer and Miss Sally Archer Anderson the need for an organization to support the nurses. The original purpose of the circle was to improve the condition of the nurses' quarters, then located on the third floor of the Hospital at 1008 East Clay Street. Those quarters were badly in need of renovation and were inadequately furnished. The Nightingales refurbished and maintained the quarters "and raised the morale of the nurses."

In 1932 the Benjamin Watkins Leigh House was presented as a gift in honor of Frances Branch Scott by her brother, Frederic W. Scott, a member of the board of directors. This building, which had served as the home of U.S. Senator Leigh, became known as Scott Memorial and the Nightingales raised money to help with its furnishings and maintenance. Various projects, such as card parties, teas, raffles, and for quite some time, the "Dance Review of the Misses Traylor and Boyle," were to benefit the work of the Nightingales at Sheltering Arms. The Tray-Boy plays were presented from 1919 to 1936, usually at the Strand Theatre.

During the presidency of Mrs. John B. Swartwout, Sr., her concern about the "impermanent nature" of the Nightingales' work led the group to endow a room in the Hospital for $10,000. By dint of hard work they produced the needed funds by 1923, and the room became known as "The Florence Nightingale Room."

In the early years the circle sewed, mended, made layettes and "dummy dolls" for nurses' training, gave yards of linoleum and gallons of paint, and more than once painted the Hospital and nurses' residence inside and out. During the Second World

War, thirty-seven members and friends of the circle helped in the Hospital because of the shortage of nurses.

Beginning with Thanksgiving 1948, school children in the Richmond area donated food in decorated baskets to Sheltering Arms. The Nightingales arranged, sorted, and stored the food when it arrived.

In 1954 when Natalie Curtis, superintendent, and Hazel Hill, assistant superintendent, retired from Sheltering Arms after thirty-two years of service, they were invited to become honorary life members of the circle. After their deaths the Nightingales established the Hill-Curtis Scholarship in 1982, in their memory, to be awarded annually to qualified student nurses.

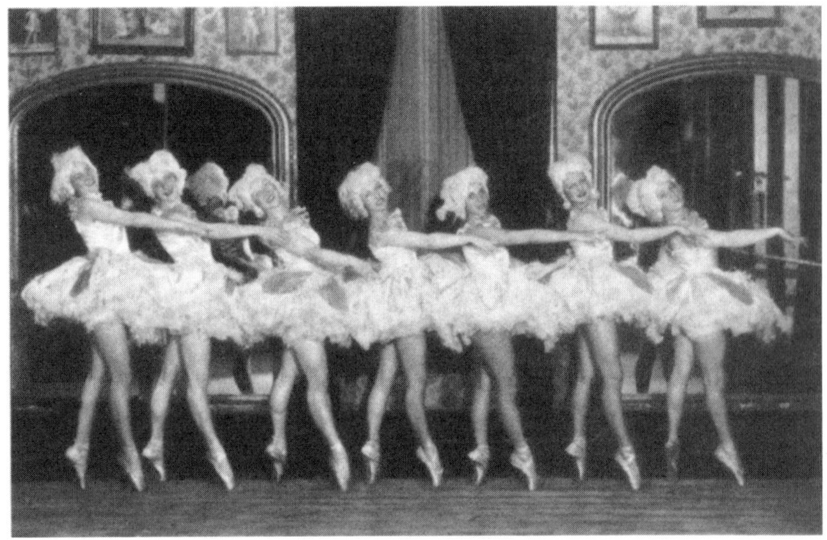

Dance reviews produced by the Misses Traylor and Boyle were a fund raising project of the Florence Nightingale Circle for many years.

Over the years, the circle has given money for improvements to the Hospital's building and facilities by providing an elevator at Clay Street, fully equipping a hospital room, and giving operating room equipment, as well as kitchen equipment, a telephone system, a blood transfusion machine, an electric bassinet, and a sun room for children. Since 1968 the annual Champagne Luncheon Fashion Show, "Fashion Futures by Thalhimers," has become the circle's major benefit project for

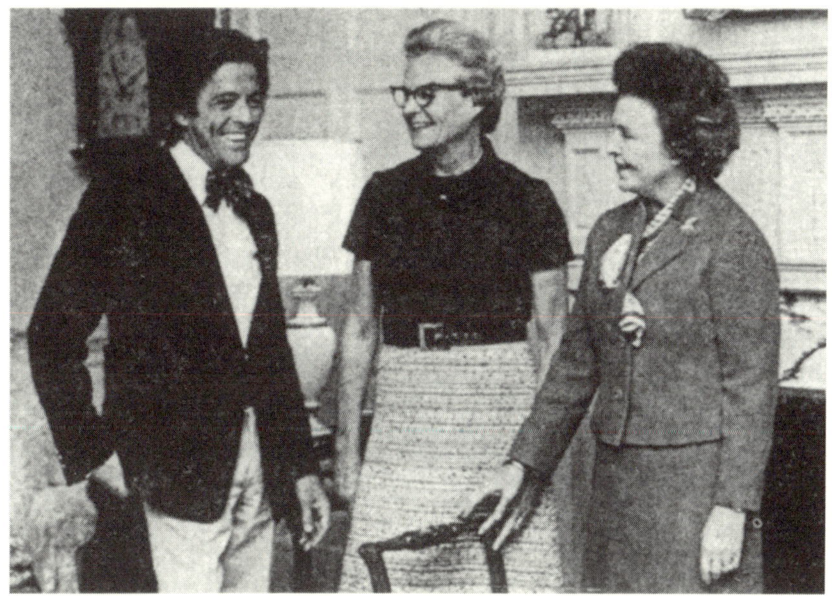

The Florence Nightingales' major benefit for the Hospital, the Champagne Luncheon Fashion Show, has produced thousands of dollars to buy equipment for Sheltering Arms. Here, fashion designer Leo Narducci shares a happy thought with Mrs. Clyde Ratcliffe, Jr., chairman, and Mrs. Mills E. Godwin, Jr., honorary chairman (1974).

Sheltering Arms. These events have contributed toward the purchase of electromyography equipment, audiology equipment, a hand-controlled driver education car, a mini-bus and a van. The circle's centennial gift to the Hospital was the state's first Regys I functional electrical stimulator (FES) for patients with spinal cord injuries.

Almost from their founding as a circle, the Nightingales would visit patients, bearing gifts and flowers. This practice evolved into a "hospitality cart," which members would bring on visits to patients' rooms. The cart, given to the circle in the early 1970s by the brother of a Nightingale in memory of their mother, was laden with toilet articles, stationery, and books. Use of the cart was discontinued during the Hospital's renovation, but resumed later as the "Patients' Comfort Cart," which the Nightingales now offer weekly in the Hospital dining area.

The words of long ago hold true: "When Sheltering Arms has a need, the Nightingales sing." After seventy-nine years of service, the Nightingales continue to sing more harmoniously than ever.

CHAPTER 6

❦ ❦ ❦

BLANCHE OLVILLE TAYLOR KING (1865-1938)

"A saint is someone the light shines through."

ONE OF THE MOST DILIGENT WORKERS in the Lord's vineyard was Mrs. George T. King, who was recorded in memory and ledger as the tireless treasurer of Sheltering Arms Hospital for forty-eight years. Born in Henrico County in 1865, Blanche Taylor was the granddaughter of William Shippen Taylor, who owned Taylor's Hill, now Richmond Hill. As a young woman she married George Thomas King, and as a member of St. James's Episcopal Church, she was one of the "handful of girls" encouraged by Rebekah Peterkin to establish a free hospital in Richmond.

It must have been a busy life in the 1890s, even by today's standards. In 1892, when the first executive board was founded, young Mrs. King was actively involved. That same year, she bore her youngest child, George; she already had a stepdaughter, Rena, and a daughter, Blanche. Mrs. King was treasurer on the new board, and carried out her duties with loving devotion and steadfast attention to detail until her death in 1938.

"You know," says her daughter-in-law, Mary O'Bannon King, "those women did everything, including scrubbing floors." "Mother King" went almost daily to Sheltering Arms to do the account books. There were times when the bank balance neared zero, yet she wrote out the salary checks, to the consternation of her son George who commented, "Mother, you have written checks for the hospital salaries without enough money in your bank account!" "Well, that's all right, George," she replied. "I am going home to pray about it." And somehow the donations came in to keep the treasury solvent. Faith seemed to multiply good work so that there was enough to spare.

What an accolade Mary King gives her mother-in-law: "I never knew her to be sad; she was always optimistic." As Mrs. King made known her faith that the Lord would send help, the

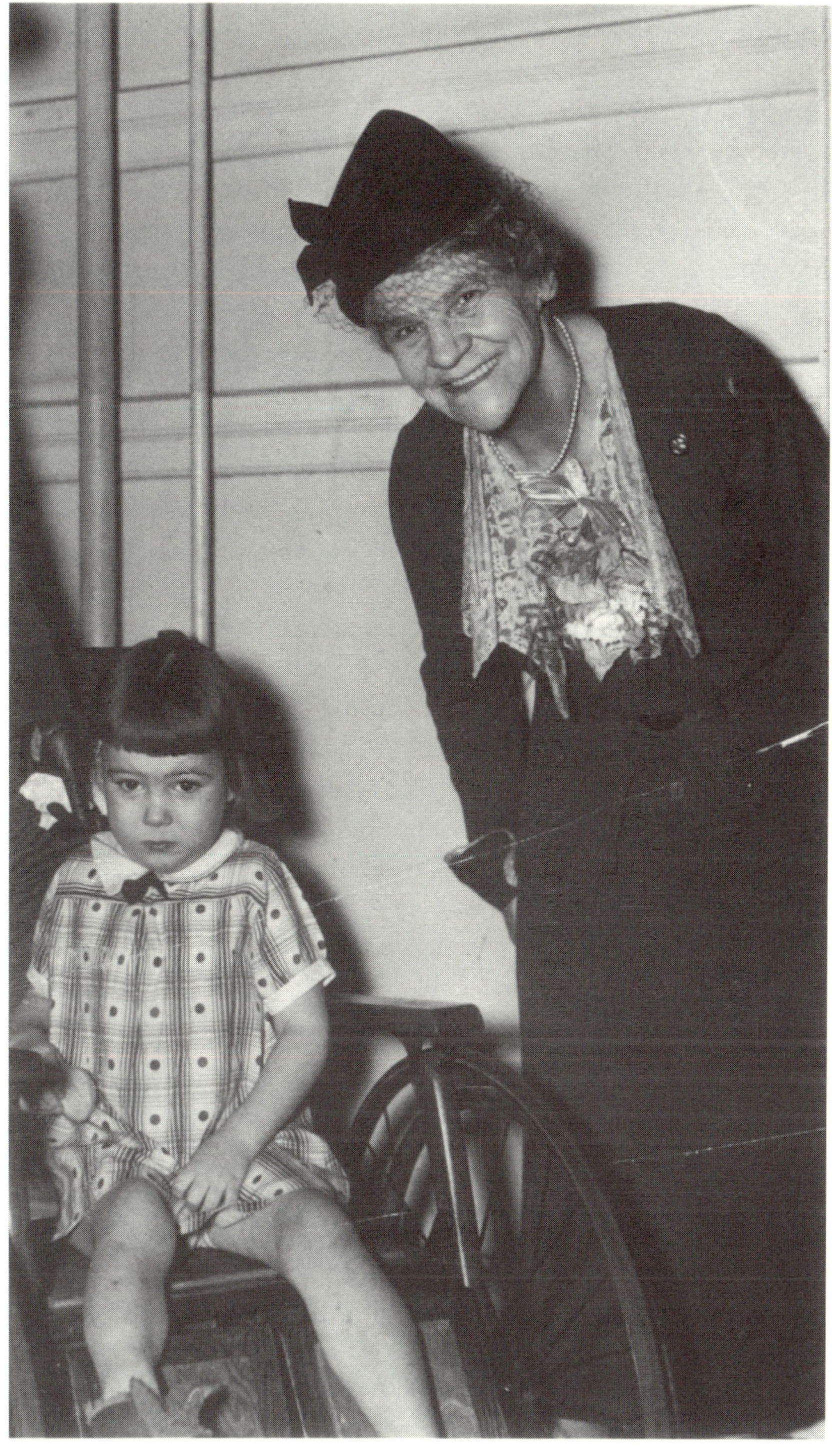

Full of godly wisdom and good cheer, Mrs. King was a diligent and almost daily worker at the Hospital. One of her favorite verses is inscribed over the entrance: "Behold what God hath wrought."

number of friends of Sheltering Arms grew, the bills were paid, and the Hospital expanded.

Eda Carter Williams describes this remarkable woman as combining the qualities of a shrewd financier with the faith and zeal of a missionary. For nearly half a century as treasurer, Mrs. King adhered to a pay-as-you-go plan: as the hospital treasury was depleted, the number of patients had to be curtailed until monetary help was forthcoming. And we know that Sheltering Arms did not want to turn patients away.

For almost five decades, Blanche King exemplified Rebekah Peterkin's inspiring idea to serve mankind. When she herself was in her last illness and her doctor, J. Powell Williams, had arranged for a bed at nearby Stuart Circle Hospital, Mrs. King announced, "I won't go to any hospital except Sheltering Arms. Everybody knows me there." And her children abided by her wishes. If people did not understand why she died in a charity hospital, it was because that hospital was Mrs. King's beloved Sheltering Arms. She was happy there and the staff was wonderful to her. Mrs. King was buried at Hollywood Cemetery on June 21, 1938.

In appreciation of Mrs. King's untiring and inspiring work for the Hospital, a King's Daughters circle of Sheltering Arms nurses was formed in her honor, the Blanche Taylor King Circle, and over the door of the sun parlor at the Grant House was inscribed one of her favorite verses, *"Behold what God hath wrought."*

Mrs. King had acted as president of the executive board after Miss Scott died in March 1937.

On Donation Day 1964, just before the move to Palmyra Avenue, the Richmond newspaper touted the occasion that gave *"honor to Mrs. George T. King, well deserved, for in those first years of organization and struggle, Mrs. King kept the books balanced and the lights and heat on. She made sure the coal-house was kept locked, hunted bargains in purchases of all kinds from coal to eggs, and she and another board member, Mrs. H. W. Bassett, even painted the diet kitchen in 1906 in order to save expenses."*

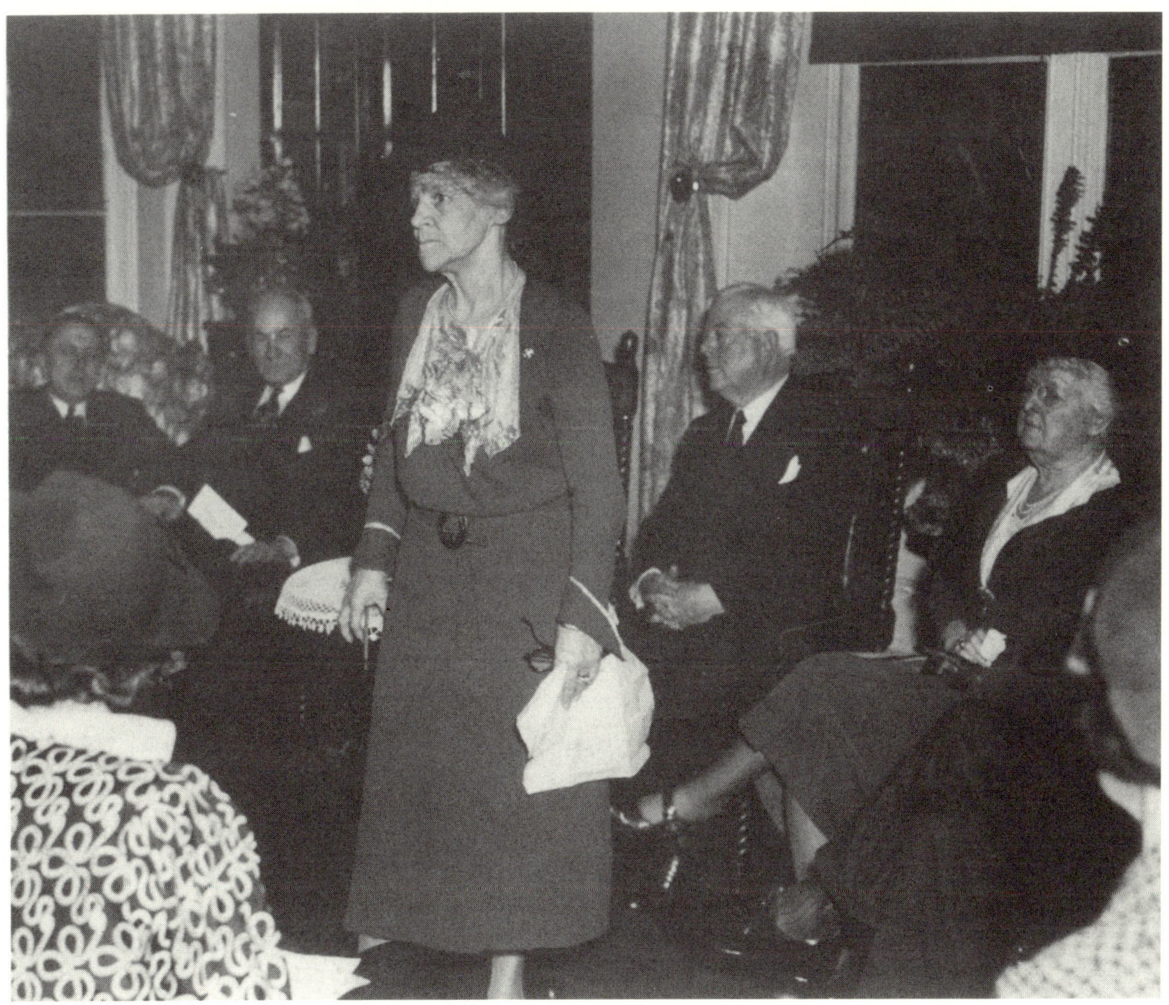

The indomitable fund raiser and faithful treasurer for 48 years, Mrs. King here gives the financial report at the 1935 annual meeting.

NATALIE CURTIS, R.N. (1889-1968)
HAZEL HILL, R.N. (1888-1977)
The Spirit of Teamwork at Sheltering Arms

SHELTERING ARMS HOSPITAL WAS FORTUNATE to have two dedicated nurses and beautiful human beings as part of its history. Their extraordinary skills and personalities so complemented each other that they must be presented as a unit to appreciate their contribution.

In the story of Sheltering Arms, Dr. Caravati praises Miss Natalie Curtis and Miss Hazel Hill as very unusual women. "I have never seen anywhere two more dedicated human beings: they believed in Sheltering Arms firmly, and believing in it, they would do anything to accomplish what they thought was the right thing. Absolutely unselfish. The wonderful thing was that whatever one of them did was all right with the other one. They never caught fire, and if they did, nobody ever knew it."

People's memories of Miss Curtis and Miss Hill are vivid, and fortunately some anecdotal material is preserved in writing from an interview of Miss Hill by Peggy Chisholm Boxley in 1955. Hazel Hill, of Columbus, Ohio, was twenty-two when she began training at the Philadelphia Orthopedic Hospital and Infirmary for Nervous Diseases in the fall of 1910. Ahead lay a long and often difficult career, dedicated to helping others. Even from the first it was not easy. Discipline was rigid. Prospective nurses at Philadelphia O & I worked twelve and a half hours' duty each day, with barely two hours' relief from their labors.

On her first day, Miss Hill's studied composure was shaken when her trunk failed to arrive and gave every sign of being lost forever. Her anxiety increased when she heard the command, "Hurry and do this, Miss Curtis won't like it if it isn't done." Obviously Miss Curtis, whoever she was, was someone to be reckoned with.

After such a discouraging start, Miss Hill became panic-stricken later that same day, when she was left to tend the children's ward alone, while the rest of the nurses went out to supper. The evening proved uneventful until suddenly all the children simultaneously asked for bedpans. As she hurried from bed to bed, she dropped one of the pans and found herself staring down at shattered fragments of white porcelain. The panic that had subsided mounted again as she thought that surely she would be dismissed from the hospital for such clumsiness. Close to tears, Miss Hill looked up to see a tall, slim, dark-haired girl of about her own age whose soft, pretty face registered a consoling sympathy. Picking up the broken pieces, the tall young nurse wrapped them in some papers and escorted Miss Hill down the hall. "You're supposed to report this," she advised, "but that won't be necessary; we'll just put this bundle in the trash and say no more about it. I broke one the first day I was here."

Thus began the friendship that carried these two stalwart nurses through decades of hard work and public service together. "Always, Miss Curtis was the executive," observed Miss Hill, "the determined, efficient one." It was she who showed

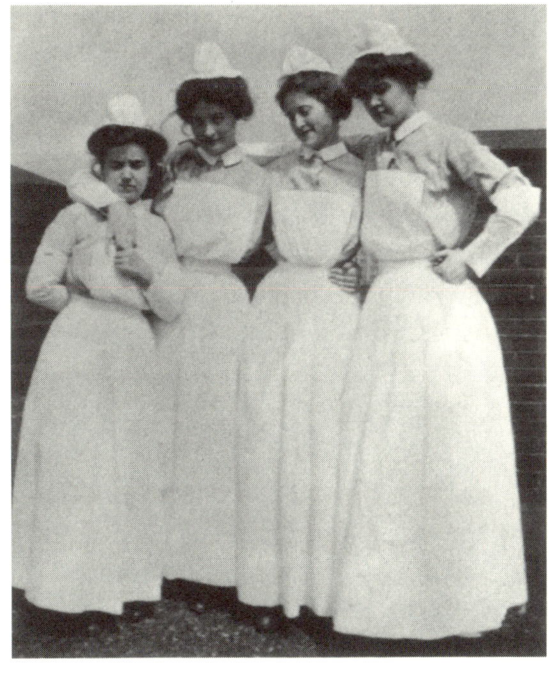

Miss Curtis (right) and Miss Hill (second from right) as nursing students at the former Philadelphia Orthopedic Hospital and Infirmary for Nervous Diseases.

the admiring Miss Hill how to clean floors by moving the cloth with her feet instead of on her hands and knees. At one point, Miss Curtis announced prophetically: "When we get through we'll work together—I'll be superintendent and you'll be head nurse." They finished nurses' training and graduated in 1913, members of the first class to complete the three-year course. Miss Hill returned to Ohio, Miss Curtis to her home in Richmond, Virginia.

Two years later, in 1915, Dr. Ennion Williams organized Richmond's first public health course. Miss Curtis, filled with enthusiasm, summoned Miss Hill from Ohio to enroll in the course with her. After six weeks of study, Miss Curtis secured a job with the City Board of Health as a public health nurse, and Miss Hill was assigned to a milk station in the basement of the Zionist Institute.

A year later, Miss Curtis' beloved father died, and Miss Hill loyally decided to remain in Richmond with her friend. The two found work at Tucker's Sanatorium, a private mental hospital in Richmond: Miss Curtis as assistant superintendent of nurses, Miss Hill as a private duty nurse. Here Miss Curtis came to the attention of Miss Ethel Smith, state inspector of nurses' training schools. Sheltering Arms Free Hospital was in urgent need of a firm, capable superintendent, and Miss Smith hoped that she could persuade Miss Curtis to take the job. After an interview with Miss Frances Branch Scott, president of Sheltering Arms' executive board, Miss Curtis accepted the position in 1922, becoming the thirteenth superintendent of Sheltering Arms. At that time the Hospital was badly disorganized. A series of superintendents had left it in a state of weakened administration; understaffed and poorly equipped, it was not even accredited.

When Miss Curtis assumed her duties, there were only three graduate nurses, nine student nurses, no interns, and no instruments in the operating room. Upon arrival the first day she was greeted by a nurse dressed in street clothes holding two large rings of keys; the other two nurses had already left. She handed Miss Curtis the keys and departed, leaving the new superintendent bewildered, with no idea of where anything was or what needed to be done. Before she had a chance to explore, an ambulance arrived. The driver and a doctor jumped out and brought a woman into the Hospital on a stretcher. "See that this woman gets to the operating room," the doctor ordered. "But I don't even know where it is," Miss Curtis replied. So the doctor went up with the woman and performed an appendectomy. Miss Curtis stayed with her until she regained consciousness after the operation.

Desperate for help, Miss Curtis called upon Mrs. Mae Perdue Brown, a graduate of Tucker's, to work with her until she found her way around. What they found was depressing.

But it was not poor housekeeping alone that was Miss Curtis' greatest challenge. Her main problem was to get the nine student nurses trained and to have the school reinstated as an accredited institution. One night soon after she began at the Hospital, Miss Curtis found all the student nurses sitting disconsolately on the front steps waiting for the doctor who was their nursing instructor. "He's always an hour late," one of them told her. When he finally did arrive, Miss Curtis reproached him for keeping the girls waiting. "I'm a busy man," he snapped. "Yes, sir," she replied, "and therefore we won't need to take up your time anymore." "That," she claimed later, eyes twinkling, "was the most surprised man you ever saw."

Faced with the problem of teaching the student nurses herself, as well as running the Hospital, Miss Curtis was in further need of help. Of course she had someone in mind: who else but Miss Hill, whom she had tried to persuade to accompany her to Sheltering Arms in the first place. Miss Hill, however, felt that since she had been trained for specialization in the treatment of nervous diseases, she would be of more use at Tucker's. Although she finally agreed to take up new duties at Sheltering Arms, she insisted upon working a month without pay until she thought she had learned enough new skills to be worth her wages.

With Miss Hill now working at Sheltering Arms, Miss Curtis knew she had someone upon whom she could depend. "You will have charge of the nurses, the delivery room and the operating room," she said. Miss Hill was astonished at the assignment, but rose to the challenge. She was a remarkable technician, as well as an exemplary nurse. For all her years at Sheltering Arms Miss Hill gave the anesthesia in the operating room, by drip ether, and never lost a patient.

Together the two nurses began the task of putting the old Hospital back on its feet. They worked ceaselessly, taking turns doing night duty, since there was no night supervisor, and teaching the student nurses, in addition to their regular administrative duties. Miss Curtis taught the class in practical nursing, and Miss Hill instructed in five other courses. Miss Curtis persuaded the Florence Nightingale Circle to provide teaching equipment, and was soon supplied with "everything but the bones." Ever resourceful, she traded a quart of whiskey that a patient had left at the Hospital for a "bag of bones" from an orderly with one of the other Hospitals, and set to work assembling the skeleton. Both Miss Curtis and Miss Hill spent their few spare moments studying to keep one jump ahead of their classes.

In the meantime, Miss Hill set to work locating equipment for the operating room. She solicited contributions from the doctors who were donating their services at the time, and instituted a "cuss bank": profanity in the operating room was punishable by a 25-cent contribution to the instrument fund. A substantial sum was raised through this method alone. Miss Hill recalls that when one doctor, who was given to swearing in the face of unusual difficulty, took one look at the condition of a rather obese patient before him, stalked silently over to the "cuss bank" and deposited ten dollars before starting the operation.

The number of graduate nurses slowly increased, the more pressing problems began to be solved, and Miss Curtis turned to the task of the Hospital's accreditation. Charts were kept, patient records were compiled and filed, and the physician

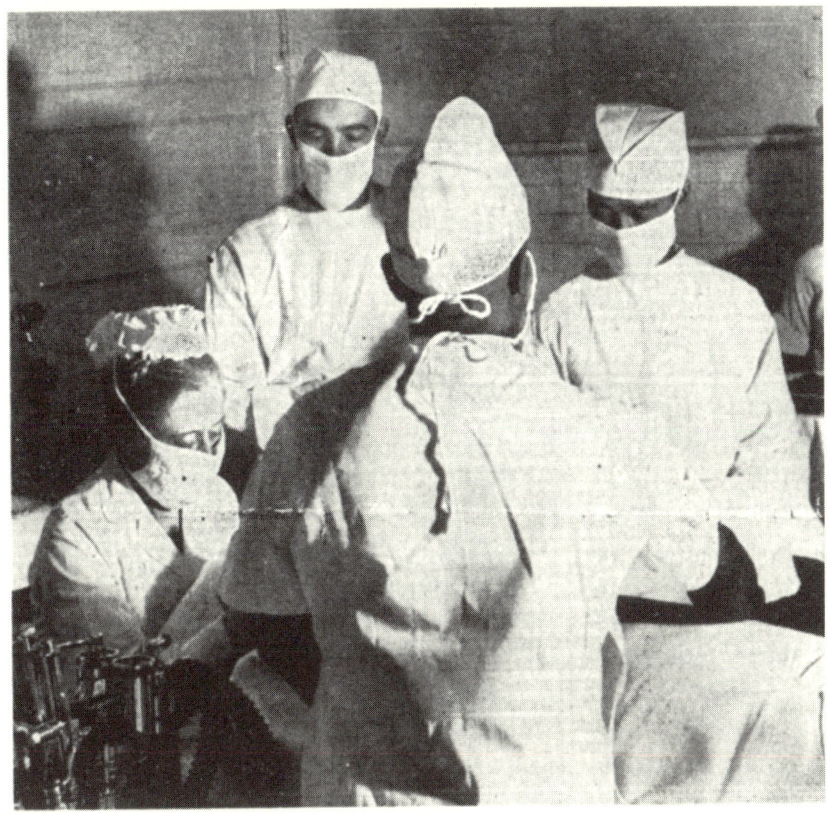

From 1922 until her retirement in 1954, Miss Hill administered anesthesia by the drip ether method without losing a patient.

staff began to hold regular meetings at the Hospital each month. The nursing school was approved, the Hospital was inspected, and finally, in 1926, Sheltering Arms was accredited.

The organizational ability that ruled the lives of these two nurses even began to penetrate the volunteer activities. Members of the Hospital's General Board and of the various auxiliaries were startled by the changes taking place. At first they were frightened by such revolutionary innovations as visiting hours and the strict rules and regulations Miss Curtis imposed. Each volunteer had always worked independently, until Miss Curtis tactfully suggested the formation of committees to take care of specific tasks. The volunteers soon discovered, however, that for all her system and efficiency, Miss Curtis would sometimes have to call for help, and when she did, no one ever turned her down.

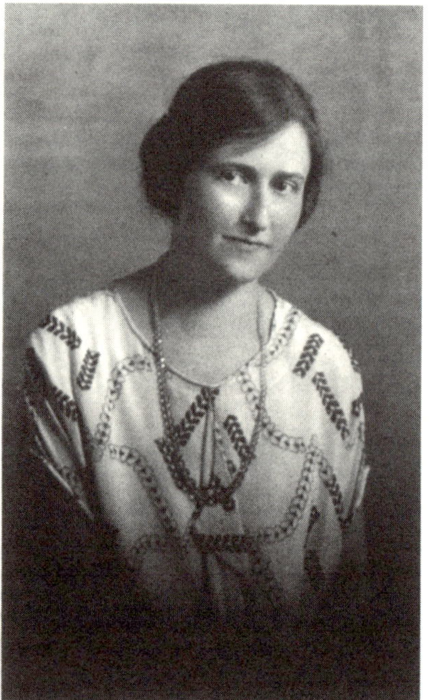
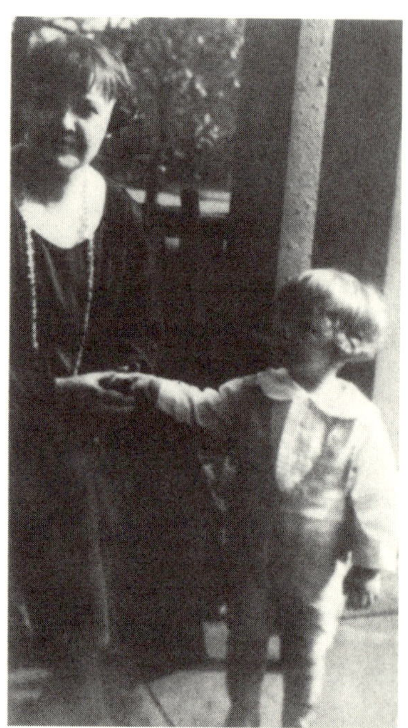

Miss Hill (left) and Miss Curtis (right), with her adopted son, Tommy.

Around 1923, about a year after Miss Curtis came to Sheltering Arms, a three-month old infant boy named Tommy was brought in as a patient. The tiny baby weighed less than six pounds; no one thought he could live. Although another hospital had refused to take him, Miss Curtis accepted him and immediately called in a young pediatrician. Tommy had been at Sheltering Arms six months when it was discovered that his mother was dying of tuberculosis. His father seemed willing to find someone to adopt him, and when Tommy was a year old, Miss Curtis decided to do so herself. "Everyone at the hospital was fond of him already," Miss Hill explained. "He had adorable eyes that looked up at you and talked."

Tommy lived at the Hospital, where he would play with another child, Joe Turpin, the son of a Negro couple who worked at Sheltering Arms. Tommy and Joe shared a black puppy. "Curt," as Tommy called his new mother, put swings and a sandbox in the nurses' yard for them. Another of Tommy's friends was "Cooper," a hunchbacked child who was a patient at the Hospital.

To Miss Curtis, Tommy was probably the most important patient ever to enter the Hospital, but her sincere interest in all the patients kindled a unique spirit at Sheltering Arms. For a lonely old man she baked a birthday cake. With the help of Miss Hill, board members and others, she arranged a Christmas party, complete with stockings and gifts, for the children confined to the Hospital during the holidays. Throughout the Depression countless people were fed from the Hospital's kitchen and many others had occasion to remember and acknowledge the kind treatment they had received. Former patients have expressed their gratitude in many ways: one farmer came into Miss Curtis' office a year or so after his discharge with a bag of pennies carefully saved to repay in some small way the care he had received at Sheltering Arms. Others contributed in goods and services what they could not give in cash. Sheltering Arms became known as "the hospital with a heart."

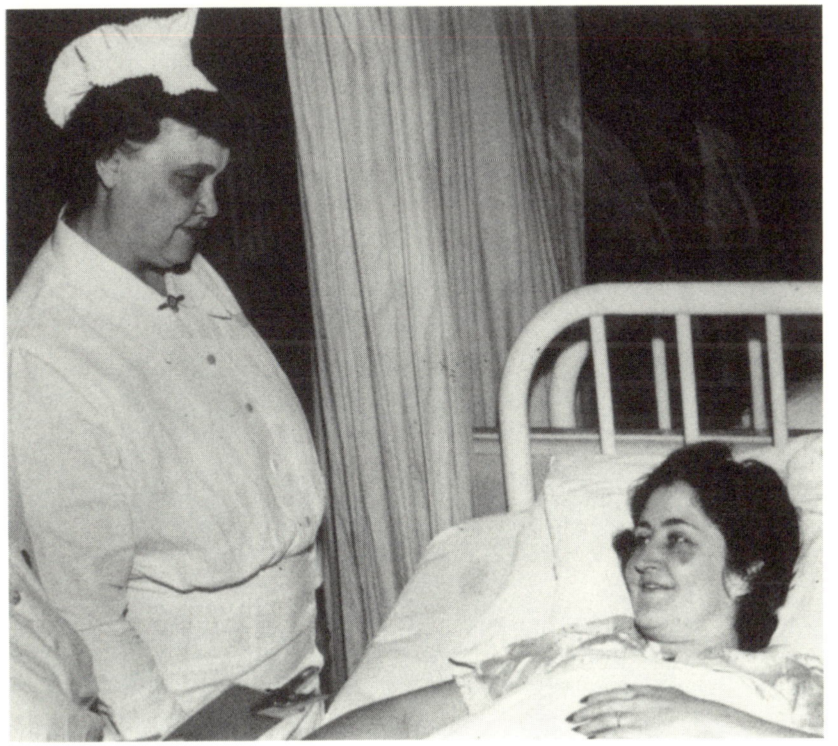

Throughout her long tenure as superintendent, Miss Curtis' main concern was for the welfare of the patients, who responded with gratitude and loyalty to the Hospital.

Throughout the years, Miss Curtis solved not only the Hospital's major challenges but also its smaller problems, with ingenuity and humor. She did a little of everything everyday, from repairing the furnace to locating suitable clothing in which to bury a destitute patient who had died at the Hospital. One small incident illustrates Miss Curtis' resourcefulness. A flock of starlings had taken up residence at Sheltering Arms and proved such a nuisance that Miss Curtis determined something had to be done. Having tried everything else without success, she finally thought of setting off giant firecrackers to scare them away. The use of firecrackers was illegal in the city of Richmond, so Miss Curtis called the Police Department and explained her plight, asking if they knew of any way to get rid of the birds. "No," said the sergeant. "Well," said Miss Curtis, "I have heard of one way, but. . ." "Lady," said he, "don't tell me a thing

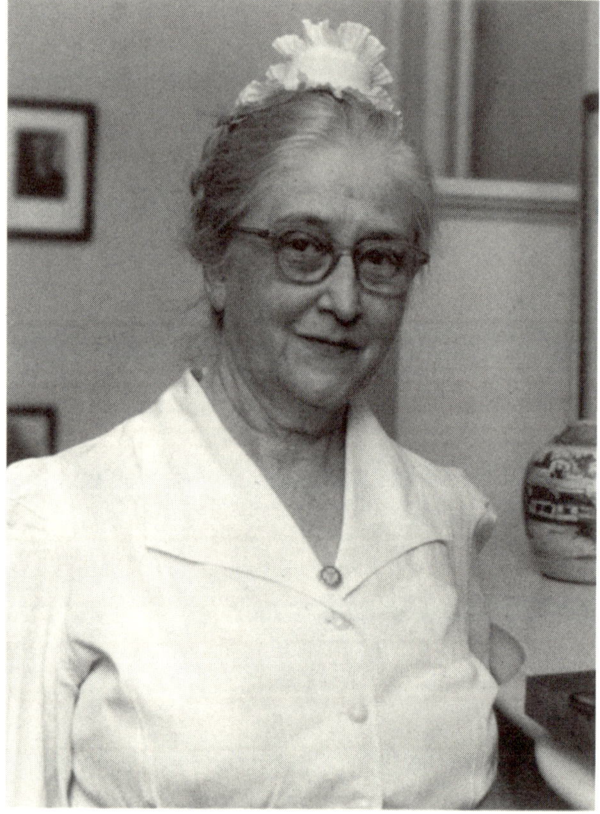

For 32 years, Miss Hill (left) and Miss Curtis (right) worked as a team in expressing their dedication to Sheltering Arms: they organized and led the Hospital and nursing school to accreditation; they inspired doctors and lay people to donate their services; and they responded to the individual needs of each patient.

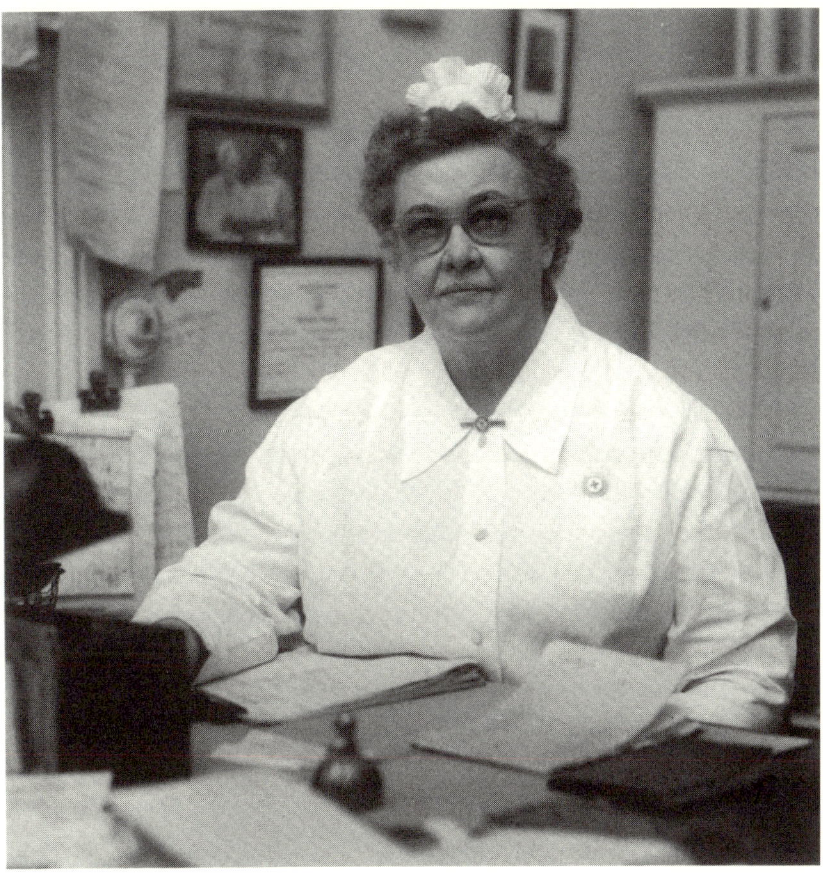

about it.'' ''Very well,'' replied Miss Curtis as she hung up, and immediately sent someone to the roof to explode the ''baby-wakers,'' as they were called. After two or three explosions, the starlings left their roost. Later, Miss Curtis was often asked how she did it, but she could not share her secret solution.

The resolution of minor crises, interesting though they may be, fades into insignificance when one considers the monumental achievement of these two nurses. Not only did Miss Curtis and Miss Hill restore the order and efficiency so necessary to the Hospital's effectiveness, but by their dedication inspired others to follow them. The positive atmosphere they created, the good morale, and the belief in the value of what they were doing, won for Sheltering Arms widespread public affection and esteem.

In 1951, Miss Curtis, a devout Roman Catholic, received a citation from the Pope in recognition of her work at Sheltering Arms. But if such work could not have been achieved without her own determined, efficient leadership, neither could her successes have been realized without Miss Hill's quiet, loyal support and devoted service. In her unobtrusive way, Hazel Hill contributed as much to the spirit of the Hospital as did Natalie Curtis. As a team they filled Sheltering Arms with a sense of unity and importance and service gladly given, and together they retired from service to the Hospital on December 31, 1954.

Following their retirement both Miss Hill and Miss Curtis volunteered as nurses' aides at MCV, making beds and doing all the important "little things" to make patients comfortable. They lived in the home they had shared on Monument Avenue until Miss Curtis' death in 1968. Miss Hill continued her contact with Sheltering Arms, and would have given the opening prayer for Donation Day 1977, but was killed in an automobile accident before the event took place. Both are buried in St. Joseph's Cemetery in Petersburg.

❦ ❦ ❦

LAURA MARIA VIETOR, R.N. (1890-1981)

"Honor, Truth, Love: Cornerstones of Nursing."

THE NURSE WHO SAID THOSE WORDS, Laura Maria Vietor was born in Bon Air, an old resort community across the James River from Richmond. She grew up on a farm where Willow Oaks Country Club now stands, and later moved with her family to a new home on Riverside Drive, which she shared as an adult with her sister Elisabeth. Their father was a successful tobacco exporter.

Laura was first educated at home by her aunt, Fraulein Graeber, who was a strict disciplinarian and an exacting teacher. In 1901 she entered Miss Jennie Ellett's School, now St. Catherine's School in Richmond. She and her sister Hanna continued their education in Switzerland.

Laura Vietor's greatest ambition was to be a nurse, and toward this end she served as a volunteer at the Diakomissen Hospital in Bremen. Her parents considered nursing a difficult life for a young woman, but following the persuasive influence of their family doctor they allowed Laura to enter the Johns Hopkins University School of Nursing in 1914.

When Miss Vietor graduated in 1917 the influenza epidemic was surging through the United States and an urgent call was issued for nurses to go to the Cumberland Mountains. The dominant forces in Laura Vietor's life were her religion, her love for her church, and her desire to be of service. As Margaret McElroy later said of her in 1983, it was characteristic that Miss Vietor was among the first to volunteer to go to this remote area where the situation was desperate and where she could follow her strong convictions.

Miss Vietor returned to Richmond after the epidemic and became night superintendent at St. Elizabeth's Hospital, where she remained for five years and founded the nurses training school. Wanting to work with children, Miss Vietor spent the next four years at the Children's Home Society, until the decision was made to put the children up for adoption. Around 1928 she became head nurse at Sheltering Arms, where she remained an integral part of the Hospital's staff until her "permanent" retirement in 1965.

Trained in nursing and pharmacology at Johns Hopkins, Laura Vietor's long service at Sheltering Arms included supervision of the drug room as well as head nurse.

A paragon of nurses, Miss Vietor "was trained at Hopkins, where nurses scrubbed floors and didn't speak to the doctors unless the doctors spoke to them first," recounts Mrs. McElroy. Miss Vietor ran a tight ship and expected the nurses under her to work as hard as she did. Laura Vietor dedicated her life to being a nurse, and with her the patient always came first.

Some nursing students recall Miss Vietor moving quickly and tirelessly among her patients and up and down the stairs. There was only one elevator in the three-story building, and it was often slow. She was never far from the patients, for she lived on the third floor. When she retired in 1955 at age 65, she told the president of the Board of Managers, Mrs. John L. McElroy, that she would work as head nurse without pay; that would be "her donation to the hospital." And so she did, for another ten years.

As a trained pharmacologist, Miss Vietor voluntarily spent long hours sorting donated drugs, thereby saving the Hospital thousands of dollars for patient care. Friends remember the meticulous way she organized the drug room on Clay Street. Katy Robinson, a volunteer with Miss Vietor, described the boxes and boxes of sample drugs from doctors' offices arriving at the Palmyra location of Sheltering Arms. There, in a cubicle built for an elevator shaft, they set up the new drug room, sorting, labeling, and storing.

For her work at Sheltering Arms, Miss Vietor was selected Richmond's "Volunteer of the Year" in 1963. She also found time, after "real" retirement at age 75, to sew children's clothes for the Red Cross, for the Quakers, for her church (St. John's United Church of Christ), and for Sheltering Arms bazaars. The Red Cross nominated her for the Senior Citizens' Hall of Fame, to which she was elected shortly before her death.

Miss Vietor was an inspiration to all who knew her, and in her honor, the Women's Council of the Hospital established the

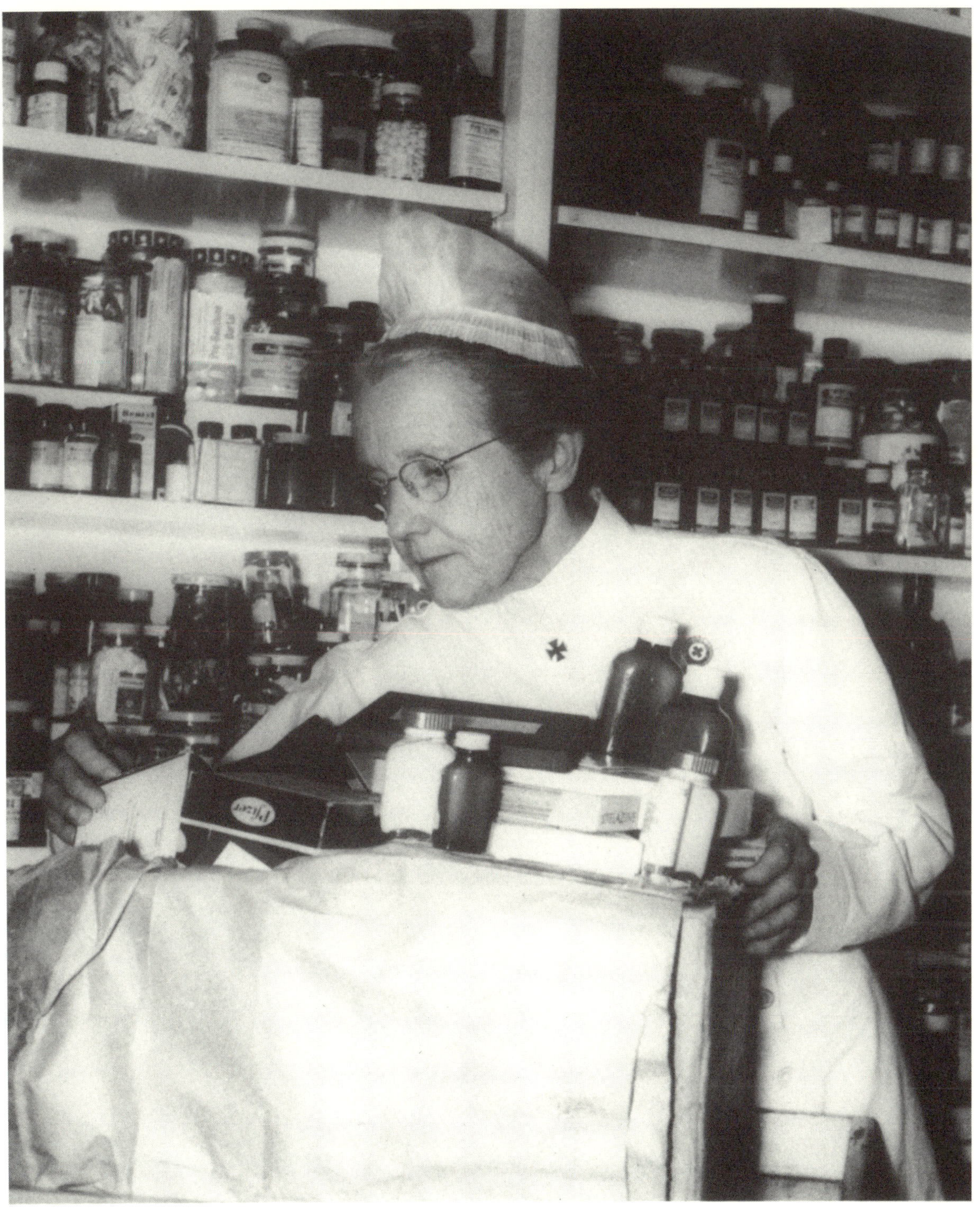

Laura M. Vietor Award for outstanding service to Sheltering Arms. "The Employee of the Year," nominated by the staff and elected by the Council, has been recognized at the climax of each Founders Day program since 1983. Recipients to date have been: Nancy Barret, Ann Stitzer, Jo Helmick, Anne Bullen, Faye Johnson, Becky Mahler, and Dee Couvelha. The award is a high honor to the employee and a living memorial to the life of Laura Vietor.

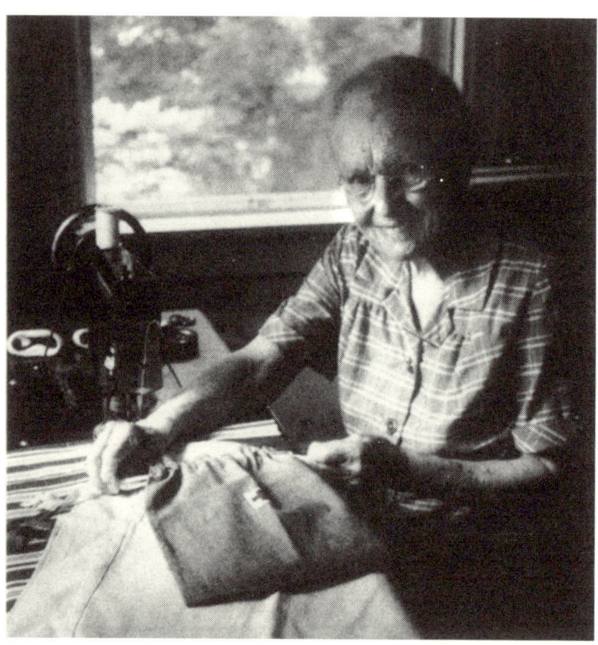

After her retirement, Miss Vietor remained active with Sheltering Arms in many ways. A member of The King's Daughters, she gave her services as a nurse for ten years without pay, and later made needed items for the patients.

❦ ❦ ❦

MARGARET NOLTING, M.D. (1887-1966)
Medical Director of Sheltering Arms Hospital, 1924-1949

THE SHORTAGE OF DOCTORS caused by the Great War of 1914-1918 directly led to a resolution by the Medical College of Virginia Board of Visitors on June 13, 1918: "Women will be admitted to the medical school because of the effect of World War I on male candidates." And thus Margaret Nolting and Mary Baughman, both of prominent Richmond families, became the first women to matriculate as four-year medical students and to graduate in the State of Virginia. Dr. Nolting took her internship at Sheltering Arms in 1922-23, and a year later became medical director of Sheltering Arms, a voluntary post she retained until her retirement in 1949. The Board elected her "honorary medical director."

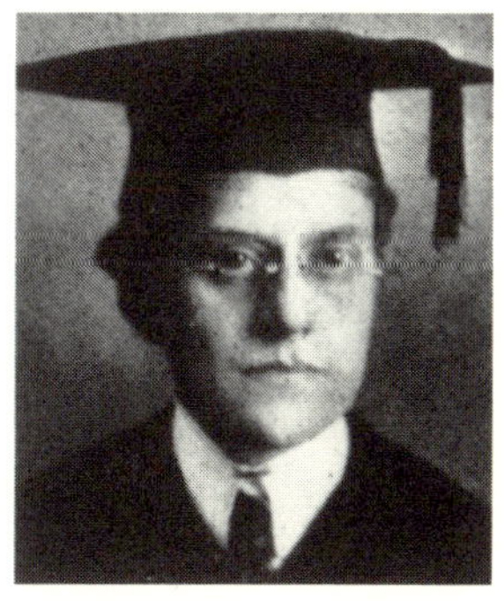

Margaret Nolting graduated from the Medical College of Virginia in 1922, one of the pioneer women doctors in Virginia.

Margaret Nolting was the youngest of twelve children of Emil Otto Nolting and Susanne Catharine Horn and lived all her life in the Nolting's beautiful family home at Fifth and Main Streets in Richmond. She attended Westhampton College during the war and returned later as physician to the students. The current president of the board of Sheltering Arms, Jean Neasmith Dickinson, Class of 1941, vividly remembers the impression this tall female doctor made upon her at Westhampton: the amazement of having a woman for a doctor and the realization that Dr. Nolting had achieved this distinction long before medicine was equally open to women.

A classmate of Dr. Nolting, Dr. Charles M. Caravati (MCV 1922), reminisces admiringly of this charming physician elected medical director of Sheltering Arms in 1924. During the next thirteen years while Miss Frances Branch Scott presided over the executive board, these two women kept an eagle eye on whether a doctor was giving good care to a patient. "I can see them now, Miss Scott and Dr. Nolting, standing on the front porch of the Hospital, conferring." If necessary, Dr. Nolting would, in no uncertain terms, reprimand a recalcitrant doctor about not seeing his patient for a few days. "As a doctor," Charles Caravati concludes, "she's the one who did more than anyone else."

Dr. Nolting was associated with St. Luke's Hospital and the McGuire Clinic in internal medicine from 1925 to 1963. A child of one of her associates there recalls this pioneer woman as being very tall and always dressed in black suits with very long skirts. But the people of Howardsville, Virginia, must remember Dr. Nolting for the great service she and Miss Courtney Irving, R.N., gave in the clinic they held in Albemarle County each summer. Memories of their "seasonal presence" there make her niece chuckle when she says, "farmers around Howardsville must have just waited to get sick until Nolting and Irving would arrive, for the patients came in droves!" Evidently, it was not uncommon that physician houseguests visiting Dr. Nolting might be pressed into service to examine patients at the clinic, and if any patients required hospitalization, they would be "carried" to Sheltering Arms by the Richmond guests or by the James River Division of the C. & O. Railroad, free of charge. One might almost call this operation "taking Sheltering Arms to the people."

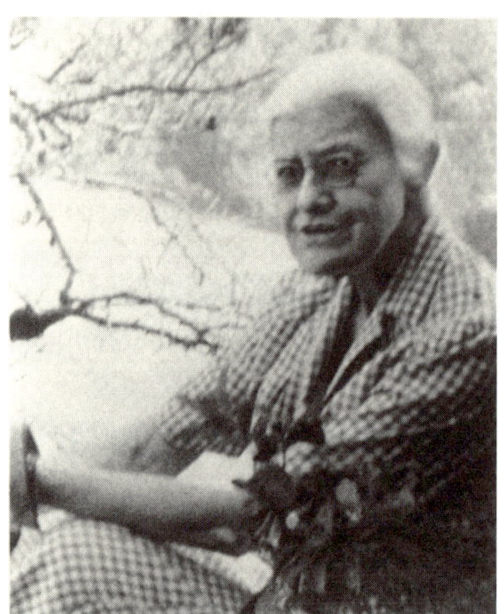

Dr. Nolting served as physician and medical director at Sheltering Arms without remuneration. After a long professional life she enjoyed another love, gardening.

FOSTER H. BERRY (1902-1979)

"The dean of orderlies"

A WISE OLD DOCTOR ONCE TOLD ME that there are two sides to medicine: the science of medicine and the art of medicine. And he went on to say that if ever there is an example of people being healed through good care, it is at Sheltering Arms Hospital. "It's the care that counts" has long been a motto of Sheltering Arms, and the prototype of tender loving care was Sheltering Arms' orderly of thirty-four years, Mr. Foster H. Berry.

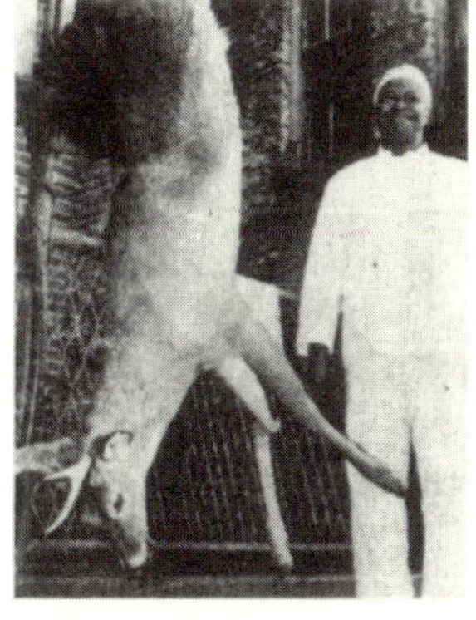

Freshly slain deer were often donated to Sheltering Arms during its years on Clay Street. Foster Berry skinned and prepared them for the cook.

His regular duties included wheeling patients to and from the Hospital operating room, turning them in their beds, helping them learn to walk again, boosting sagging spirits, and doing anything else that needed to be done. "Everyone loved Foster," said a nurse. She recalled a fire in the Hospital in 1958, caused by a clogged incinerator. "By the time I got to the third floor where the surgical patients were, Foster had already evacuated the patients, even carrying one patient in his arms down to the first floor."

His duties were mixed because Foster volunteered to do anything useful to bring comfort to the patients, even preparing food. The story is told that when a former patient gratefully brought a freshly killed deer to the back door, Foster set to skinning the deer, even though he was going off duty. "It's hard to say how many I skinned," said Foster, "but quite a few! I would take them right out behind the hospital and skin them."

And there were a few times when the man in charge of the furnace did not show up, and Foster tried to get heat upstairs to the patients. "And remember back in the war when gas was scarce? I rolled some of the patients back to their homes in wheelchairs," Foster recalled. In his "spare time" he made coffee for the other employees. Nothing was too small if it helped the Hospital. The stories are legion of this man's loving work on behalf of Sheltering Arms.

Foster Berry transferred duty to Sheltering Arms' new location on Palmyra Avenue in 1965 and continued his special attention to acute care patients until he retired in 1972, leaving with the deepest gratitude of Sheltering Arms patients and staff.

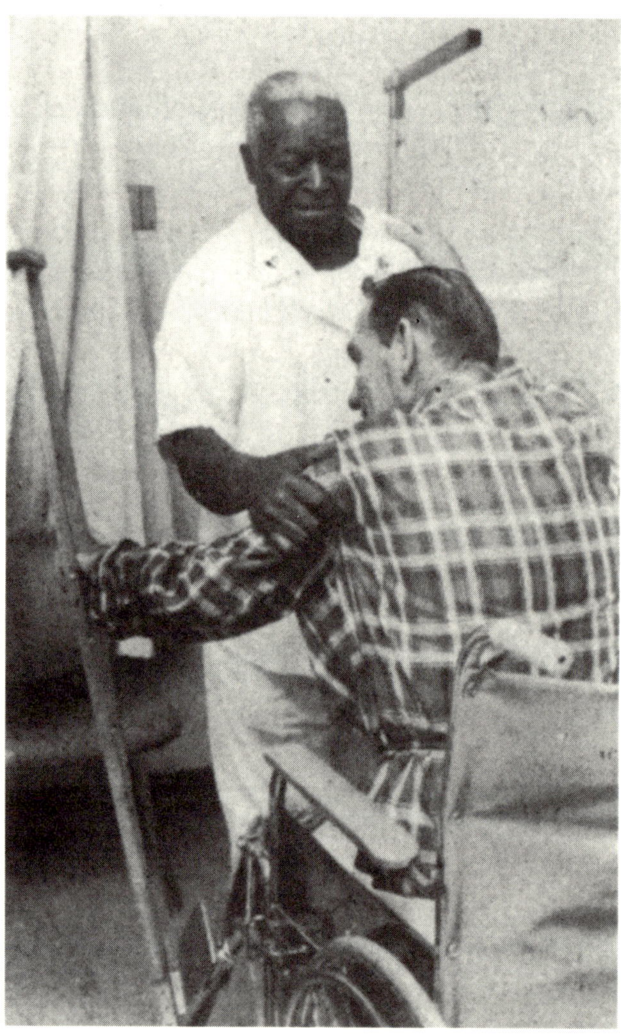

For Foster Berry, an orderly at Sheltering Arms for 34 years, no task was too large or small if it helped the Hospital or gave comfort to the patients.

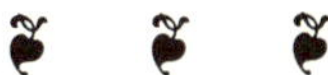

ANNE ELIZA TENNANT BRYAN (1875-1952)

"She saw all people as children of God."

FOR THE LAST FIVE OR SIX YEARS OF HER LIFE, Mrs. John Stewart Bryan attended to the little personal touches of caring for sick people and for the morale of the nurses at Sheltering Arms. Daily she was brought by car from her residence at the Jefferson Hotel to Clay Street, where she donned a white uniform and proceeded on her rounds of bringing cheer. Mrs. Bryan's visits were so eagerly awaited that one female patient is reported to have refused a nurse's offer to brush her hair, saying, "I am waiting for that lady hairdresser from the Jefferson."

Mrs. Bryan was born in Petersburg, Virginia, the daughter of David B. Tennant and Willie Anne Buffington. She moved to Richmond with her widowed mother, her sister, and her three brothers around 1895 and was educated at Mrs. Lefevre's School in Baltimore. She married John Stewart Bryan of Richmond in 1903, and they made their home at "Laburnum," where they raised two sons and a daughter. Mr. Bryan was the president and publisher of Richmond Newspapers, Inc., and was former president of the College of William and Mary, and chancellor at the time of his death in 1944. For fifty years Mrs. Bryan had been a communicant of Emmanuel Episcopal Church near "Brook Hill," and she is buried in its cemetery.

In earlier years Mrs. Bryan had devoted her time to the Belle Bryan Day Nursery where she had been president of the board. Later in life she spent part of almost every day at Sheltering Arms. Arriving laden with gifts, Mrs. Bryan worked in the wards at any task that would add to the comfort of the patients, who quite simply called her an "angel." For the nurses, Mrs. Bryan was a fairy godmother.

In the late 1940s, one board member described Mrs. Bryan as "a perfectly beautiful lady" with lovely white hair and blue eyes, tall and thin. Nothing was too humble to do for the patients. For example, when one woman who was admitted to

Sheltering Arms became distressed because she had to leave her goat unattended at home in the country, Mrs. Bryan had the goat picked up and deposited at "Goat Hill", where her son lived. She told the patient not to worry any more; the goat would be taken care of.

If a patient was discharged but had no way to go home, Mrs. Bryan sent her chauffeur to take the patient home. If a patient needed something to wear in the Hospital, Mrs. Bryan went right out to buy a pretty gown for that patient. And on hot, sweltering days, Mrs. Bryan would arrive at Sheltering Arms with three or four cases of ginger ale and gallons of ice cream for everyone.

The beautiful Laburnum, rebuilt in 1907-08 by Joseph Bryan, was the family home until 1951 when the house and grounds were given to Richmond Memorial Hospital.

Far right: A 1951 portrait of Mrs. John Stewart Bryan, a volunteer completely devoted to the well-being of patients and staff at Sheltering Arms.

For the nurses, on special occasions like graduation, Mrs. Bryan arranged a dinner party at the Jefferson Hotel with music and gifts from Schwarzschild's, personalized with the nurses' initials. "Mrs. Bryan added glamour," Miss Curtis said of these occasions. "She put glamour in our lives."

It is a friendly touch of history that Sheltering Arms should find a new home on the grounds of "Laburnum" in the 1960s. For the beautiful brick and limestone "Laburnum" had been the home of Mrs. Bryan and her family from 1908 to 1951, when it was given by them to Richmond Memorial Hospital.

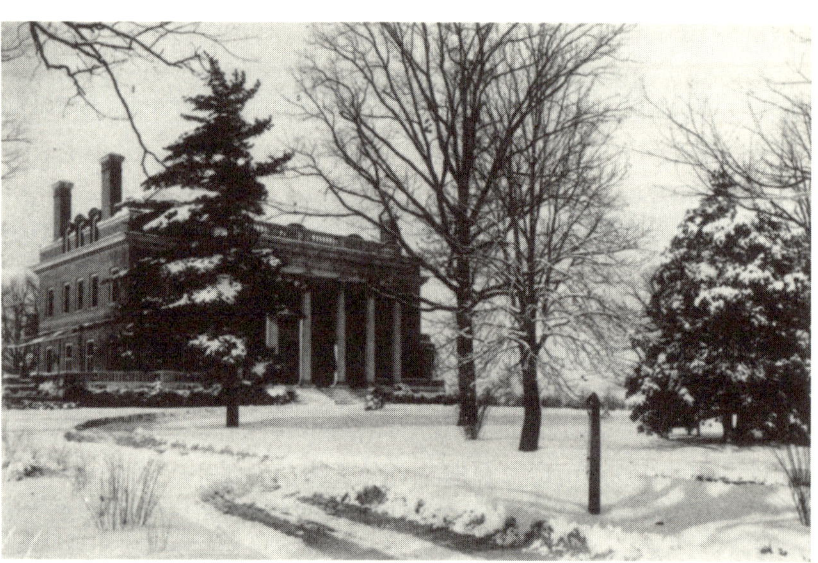

Valentine Museum

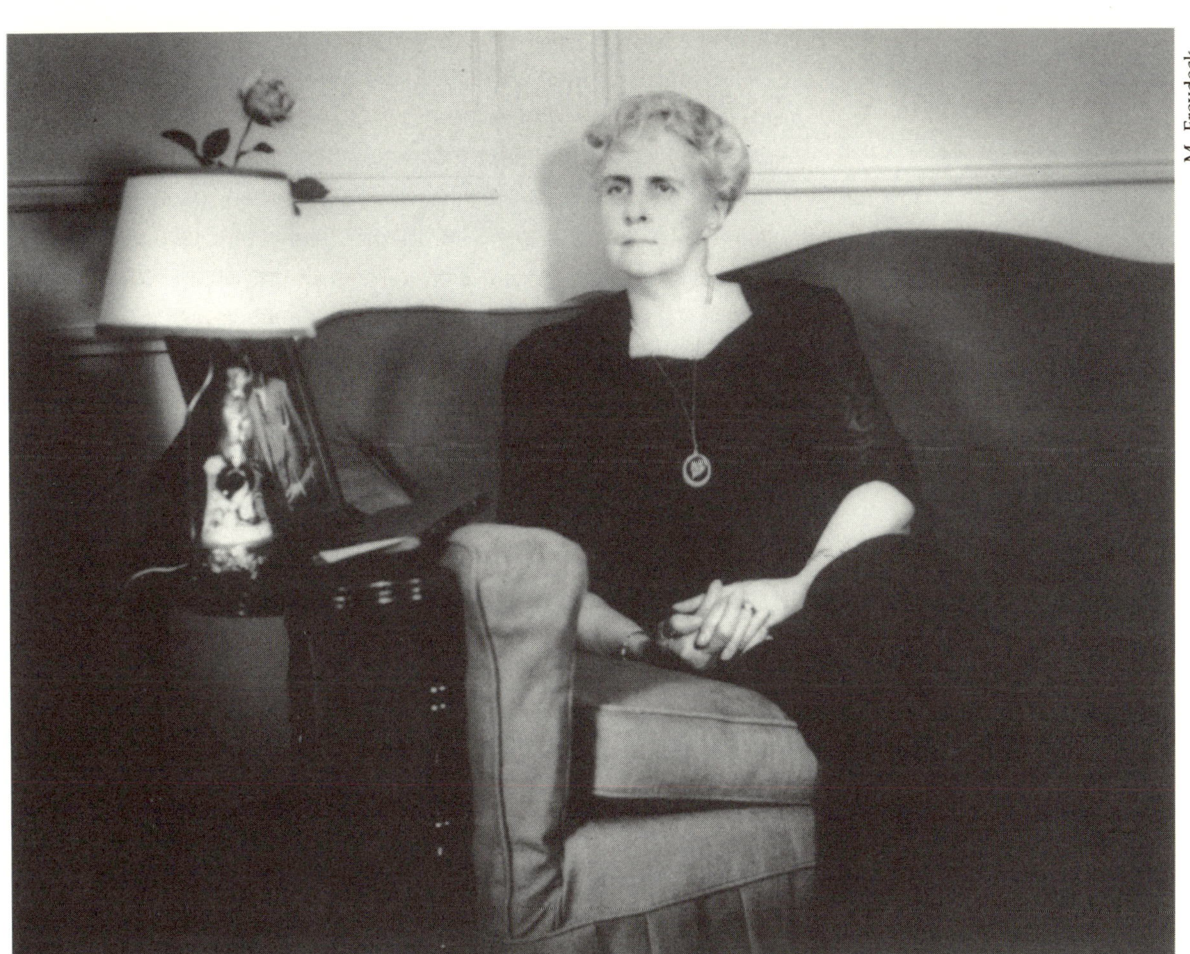
M. Freydeck

Of course, it was Mrs. Bryan's caring spirit which so inspired everyone at Sheltering Arms. In a moving tribute by Catharine Bemiss McGuire, read to the General Board on October 9, 1952, the spirit of a great lady was acknowledged:

> *It is impossible to express in words the loss which the Sheltering Arms Hospital sustained when on September 7th Mrs. John Stewart Bryan was taken from us.*
>
> *The Sheltering Arms has received many gifts from devoted and inspired friends, but the contribution of Mrs. Bryan was unique in its history. For more than five years she gave herself to this hospital.*

This gift meant to the Sheltering Arms the presence of one whose beauty, charm and character were a benediction. It meant to those working on the wards efficient help in caring for the patients and an example in doing the immediate task with enthusiasm, imagination and unselfishness. It meant to the patients the comfort of her kind and gentle care, the pleasure of her honest interest and the encouragement that only one who has shown great courage can give.

Mrs. Bryan was a happy person in that she had a clear purpose in life and perfect freedom in pursuing it. Convinced that a day not filled with service or pleasure for others was a day lost, she dedicated her time with generous energy and reckless love. To her, there were no unlovable people. She saw all people as children of God, and with almost divine perception she accepted them with pleasure, pity and patience. Those who watched her at work knew she was spending her strength beyond her resources, but she would not be stopped. She was busy planning and doing for others until the last hours of her life.

Truly the grace of our Lord Jesus Christ, the love of God, and the fellowship of the Holy Spirit were with her and we have been blessed in her association with this hospital.

THE JUNIOR BOARD

THE JUNIOR BOARD HAS BEEN SO ACTIVELY INVOLVED with work for Sheltering Arms for such a long time that no one seems to know when it actually began. One may presume that Miss Frances Branch Scott thought of asking young women to form a junior auxiliary of the executive board as a natural adjunct to the work of the older generation, which was so deeply devoted to the Hospital. Most likely, some time before 1925 Miss Scott asked the daughters and nieces of the founders and the "original incorporators" to become members of the Junior Board. Mrs. George T. King, Jr., Mrs. John L. McElroy, and Mrs. James H. Scott all recall being on the Junior Board in the mid-1920s.

Fund raising and food gathering seem to have been the primary activities of the Junior Board. At Thanksgiving time, school children contributed canned goods to Sheltering Arms. Station wagons were filled with contributions by the Junior Board, who also sorted and stored them: "potatoes over here, canned goods up there." Memories also include collecting unused food from the St. Paul's Lenten luncheons and bringing it to Sheltering Arms' dietitian, Mrs. Murphy, who carefully

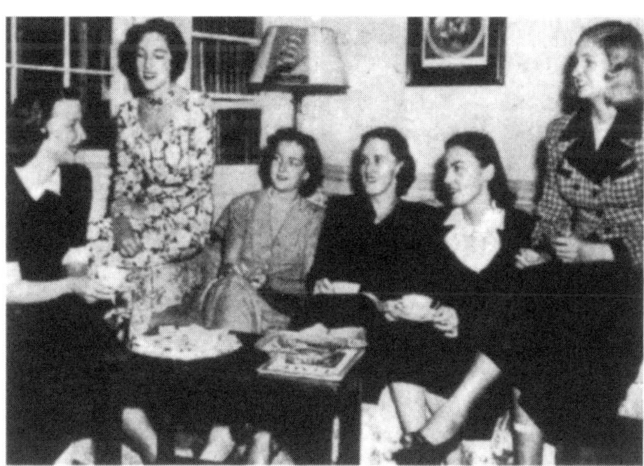

Young women who reorganized the Junior Board in 1947 (left to right): Caroline Scott, Archer Christian, Elise Anderson, Mary Stuart McGuire, Peggy Robertson, and Peggy McElroy.

prepared it for the dinner meal. At donation time, the young women were involved in folding and mailing the appeal letters.

Although Polly Scott Cardozo has a childhood recollection of selling felt pins for 25 cents at Christmas time and of visiting with Sheltering Arms patients, there seems to be no written record of the Junior Board until it was reactivated in the late 1940s. Gathered then in the McElroy living room was yet another generation of young women determined to be useful to Sheltering Arms: Elise Anderson, Archer Christian, Caroline Scott, Mary Stuart McGuire, Peggy Robertson, and Peggy McElroy. From then on stories abound of the Junior Board members who, by pairs, visited Loving's Produce and other wholesale grocers in Shockoe Slip or 17th Street Market every Saturday afternoon. These grocers gave to Sheltering Arms the leftover vegetables and fruit which could not be kept until Monday. The Junior Board delivered them via the alley behind Sheltering Arms to the basement door. Cold floors in the markets and hanging venison in Sheltering Arms' basement color the memories of forty years ago.

The Junior Board enthusiastically sought an original fund raising event for Richmond and produced the Bal du Bois, a charity ball that proved to be a smashing success. The first Bal in

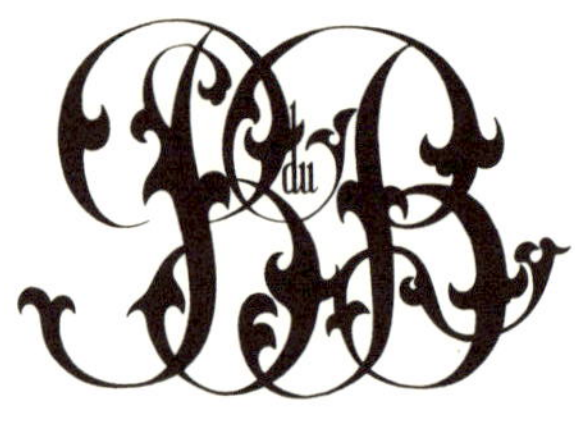

Above: Symbol of the Bal du Bois.

Far right: The Junior Board presents an annual charity ball, the Bal du Bois, which has produced thousands of dollars for the Hospital since its beginning in 1957.

Lower: Bessie Bocock Carter (second from left) was the first Bal chairman. Here (from left) with Elizabeth Hotchkiss, Robert Carter, and Mary-Louise Pinckney.

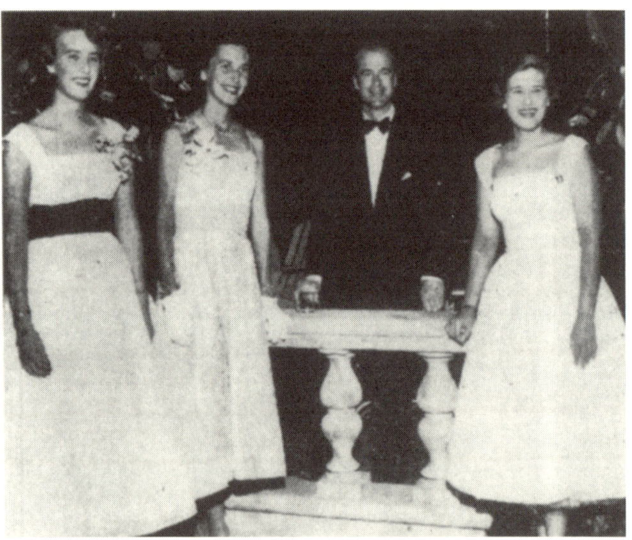

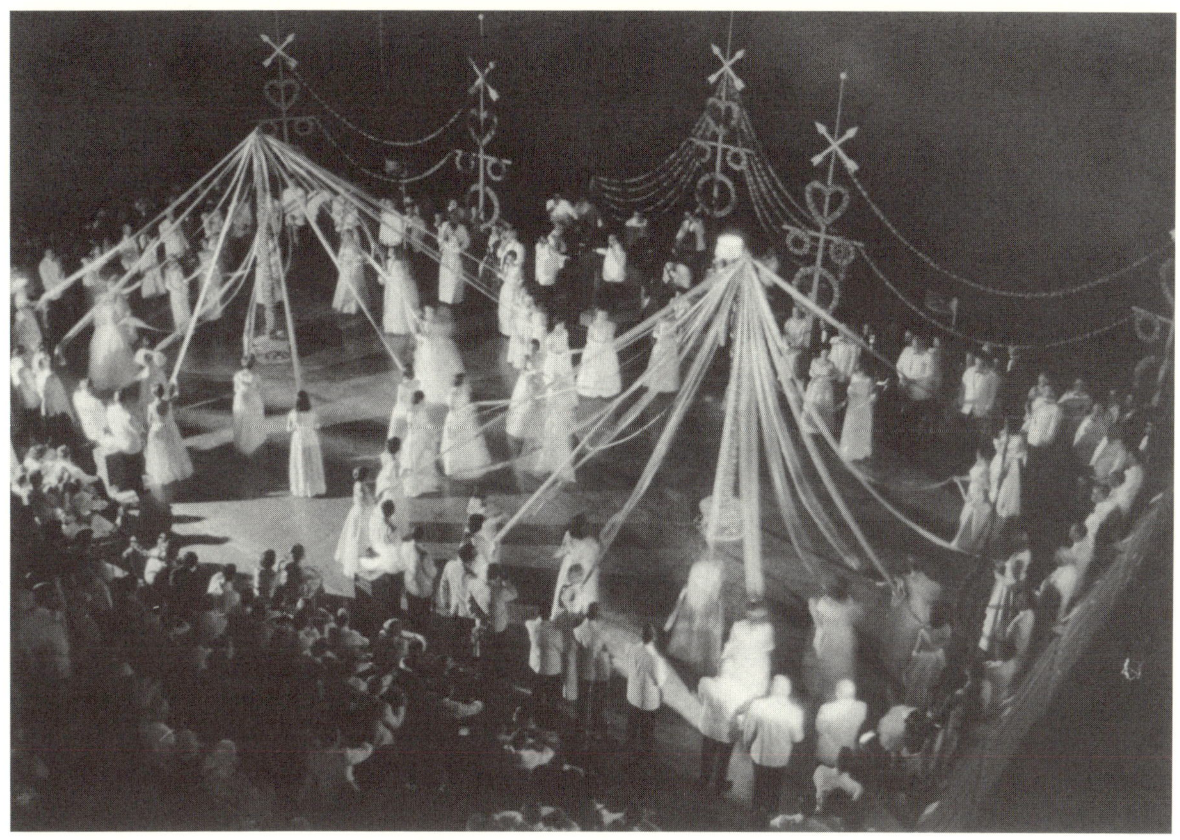

1957 was a "Garden at Versailles": a beautiful party with statuary, a fountain, and lighted chandeliers. Later, a Parisian theme followed, replete with an Eiffel Tower built by Richmond contractor Kennon Perrin.

Always an exciting part of the Bal presentation is the setting, created with the generous help of Robert Watkins and deVeaux Riddick. The young women still paint the dance floor each year, and for a long time, the elaborate scenery was painted in the alley behind the home of Mrs. Douglas Call (mother of Lucy Dabney) and stored in her garage. For years the talent of Kitty Robertson Claiborne was applied to choreographing the figure for debutantes and their fathers.

Over the years the Junior Board has done many things for the Hospital, but none so beneficial as the Bal du Bois in producing hundreds of thousands of dollars.

The Junior Board has been an integral part of the organization of Sheltering Arms and has, since the 1950s, been represented on the board of managers and its committees. Currently two past presidents of the Junior Board are directors of the Hospital, Dale Tatum Mercer and Virginia Brent Hailes.

The Junior Board's hand is always felt in their contributions to every special occasion at the Hospital, from donating baked goods for bazaars to visiting patients with valentine favors.

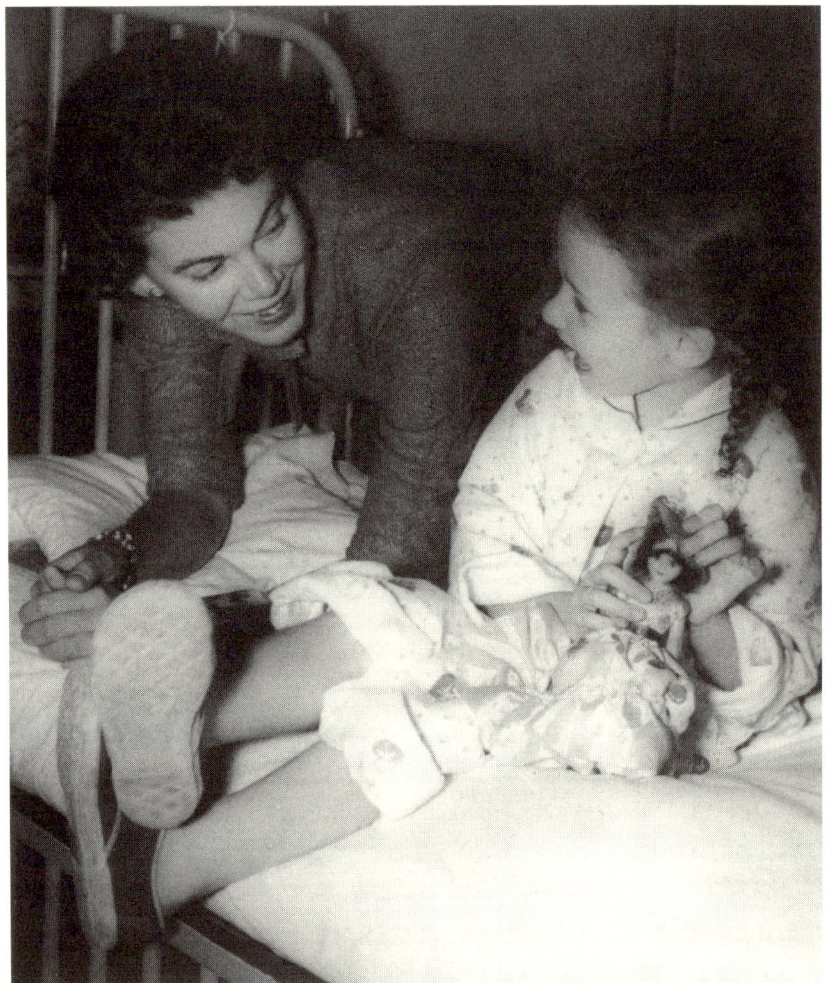

Junior Board member Mary Tennant Bryan visits children at Sheltering Arms.

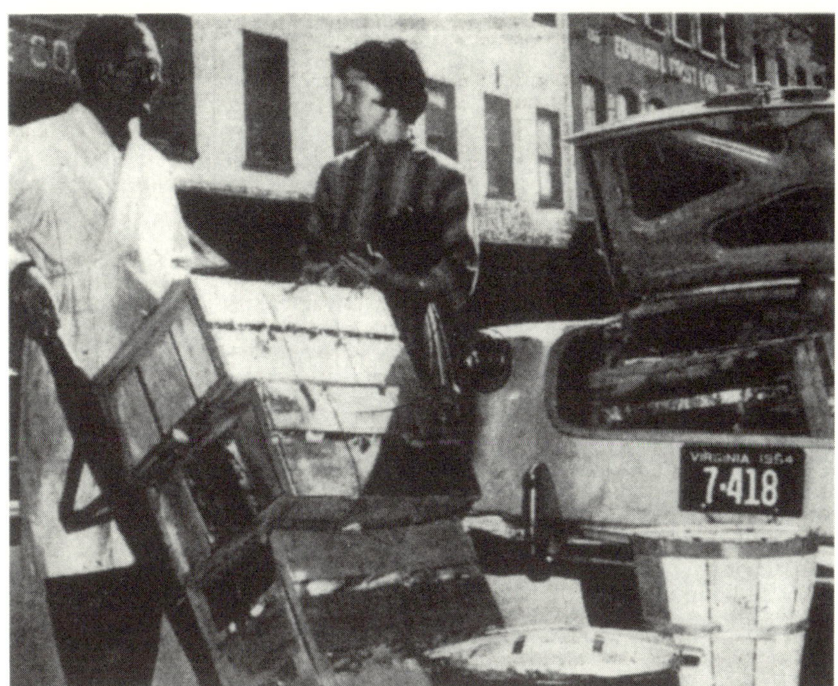

Another Junior Board member, Margaret Page Bemiss, collects fresh produce donated by a downtown market.

CHAPTER 6

BACKGROUND OF REHABILITATION MEDICINE

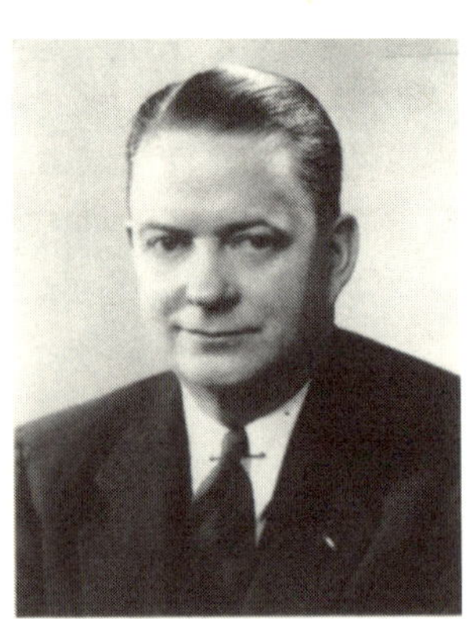

Dr. Howard A. Rusk, a pioneer in rehabilitation medicine, was the founder of the country's first rehabilitation center.

THE HISTORY OF PHYSICAL MEDICINE and rehabilitation may date back to the ancient Greeks, according to Dr. Charles H. Bonner, first medical director of the new rehabilitation hospital at Sheltering Arms. Others suggest that Dr. Simon Baruch is considered the "father" of rehabilitation medicine in the United States. Dr. Baruch graduated from the Medical College of Virginia in 1862 and, incidentally, was the father of the great New York philanthropist Bernard Baruch. In 1885 Dr. Baruch spoke of his goal of restoring patients to useful life; patients who had come to hospitals to die, only to find that with certain kinds of care, they could be partially or entirely rehabilitated. Dr. Baruch was an advocate of hydrotherapy.

The modern concept of rehabilitation, however, was developed from observations of Air Force doctors in World War II. Dr. Howard A. Rusk had learned the lessons of rehabilitation—psychological, social, and medical—from his experience with treating airmen injured in war. Lessons learned in the convalescent wards of military hospitals convinced Dr. Rusk and others that civilian patients could also benefit from the specialized care of nursing, coordinated with physical therapy, occupational therapy, psychology, speech/audiology, and prosthetics. Social services, vocational retraining, nutrition and pharmacology also added new dimensions to the patient's well-being. With self-motivation, a person could be restored to a useful life; all in spite of handicap. Activities of daily living (ADL) did not seem "medically necessary" to third-party reimbursers, but this approach, beyond traditional medicine, paid dividends in the total life of the patient.

In Dr. Rusk's rehabilitation institute at New York University in 1948, the grand experiment had taken root and soon flowered into a movement to supplement traditional departments of treatment and education. Slow to "catch on" in professional circles in the United States, physicians from abroad flocked to the young institute at 34th Street and the East River for training. They could see its application for the poor in Third World countries, as well as for victims of war in Europe.

The crusade for rehabilitation was enthusiastically carried on by lay people. Inspired by Dr. Rusk, they saw the practicality of a health care service that could rehabilitate a person disabled by disease or injury; literally, rehab could open doors to a person imprisoned in his own body. In the late 1940s, poliomyelitis was devastating a shocking percentage of American youth, and physical rehabilitation offered hope for them. Injury on the job contributed to significant lost time in a worker's life; rehabilitation addressed this problem and promoted the attitude of "adjusting" or "adapting" to a life changed by circumstance.

As rehabilitation medicine has become an accepted discipline in medical schools, there has been a concomitant growth in schools of allied health. A gradual evolution has occurred in the treatment of disability. In Richmond, Virginia, Sheltering Arms Hospital has led the way.

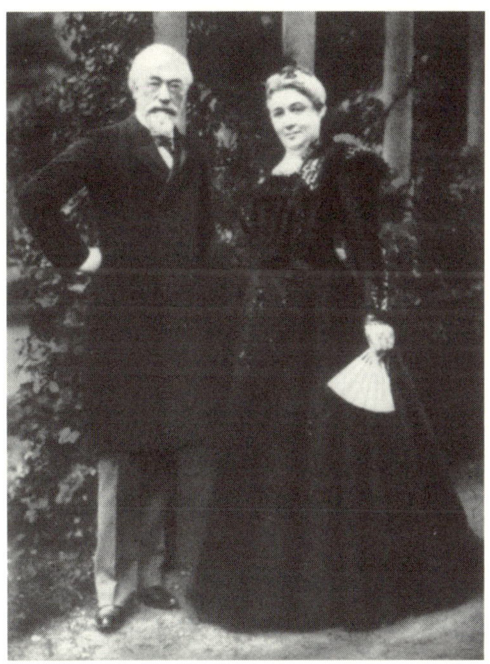

Dr. Simon Baruch, 1862 graduate of the Medical College of Virginia, and his wife. Dr. Baruch has been called the "father of rehabilitation medicine" in the United States.

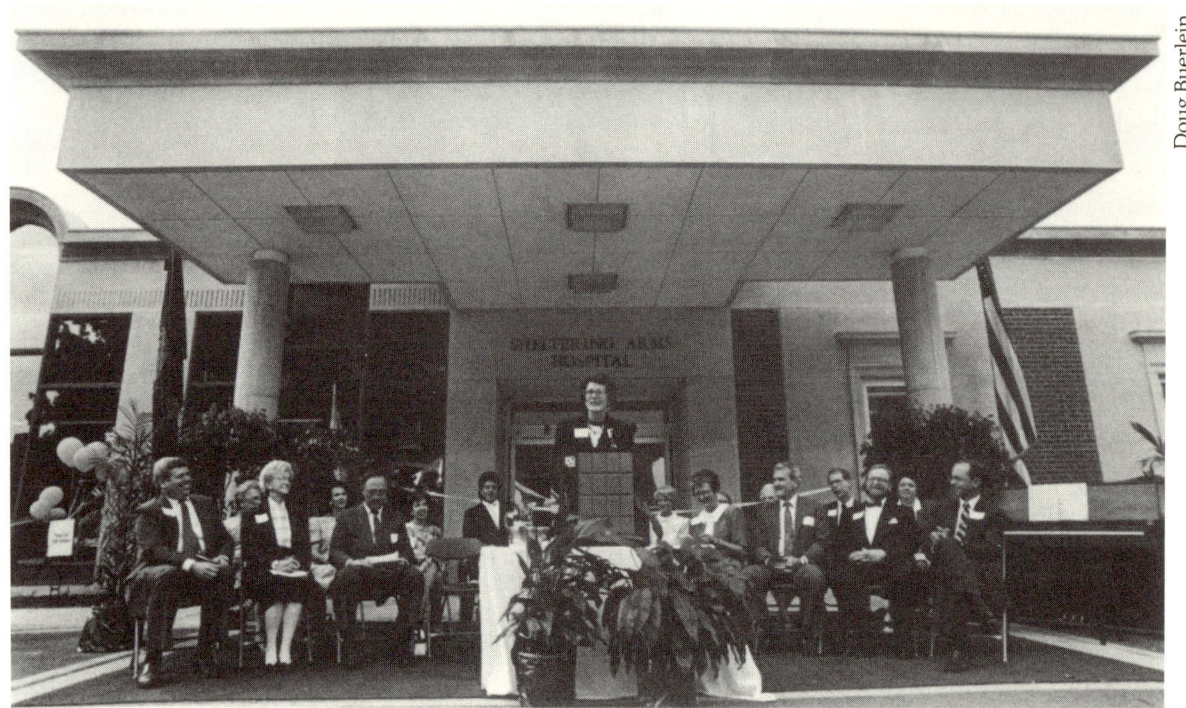

Doug Buerlein

At the Grand Opening of the new east wing in September, 1988, Jeanne P. Baliles, Virginia's First Lady, delivers the keynote address.

ACKNOWLEDGMENTS

AS THERE ARE MANY PEOPLE who make Sheltering Arms the institution it is, so there are many people who have made significant contributions to this centennial book. I would like to thank Elizabeth Herbener for research; Monica Hamm for editorial assistance; Tina Chovanec for graphic design; Joy Payne for typing; Johnnie Lou Terry for being my touchstone; Lucy Dabney and her Historical Committee of the Women's Council, and Louis Rossiter of the David G. Williamson Institute at Medical College of Virginia, for their advice. Several organizations were generous with their support of my effort: The Virginia Historical Society, the MCV Archives, the Virginia Division of Historic Landmarks, the Valentine Museum, the Beth Ahabah Archives, and the Virginia State Library.

Of people who have already given generously of themselves to Sheltering Arms and who willingly shared their experience and wisdom with me, none did so more than Eda Carter Williams. I would like to thank Margaret Williams McElroy, Peggy Chisholm Boxley, D. Tennant Bryan, Mary O'Bannon King, Nancy Kulp, Susanne Williams, Elisabeth Vietor, Dorothy Cridlin, R.N., Emma Murry, R.N., Charles Caravati, M.D., Richard A. Michaux, M.D., Milton Hobson, Keith Caudle, Thomas Curtis, Francis Booth. And two wise counselors, Mary Wells Ashworth and Virginius Dabney.

I appreciated the perspective given to me by Hunter H. McGuire, Jr., and a number of other physicians who were helpful in evaluating the role of Sheltering Arms Hospital in the Richmond medical scene.

I relished the vivid recollections of many women who had been deeply involved with the daily operation of Sheltering Arms in the years on Clay Street and would like especially to thank Ruth Thalhimer, Alice Williams Scott, Emma Gray Trigg Emory, Mary Frances Flowers, and Charlotte Massie.

ACKNOWLEDGMENTS

To draw together the threads of events and people into a one hundred year chronicle required the efforts of many individuals at Sheltering Arms. Quite simply, though, I could never have completed my work without Nancy Barret, Betsy Terrell, and Wayne Humphries.

In written material I am grateful for the help of Richmond Newspapers, Inc., and for the enlightenment of the following books:

A History of St. James's Episcopal Church, 1835-1985, edited by Margaret T. Peters.

History of the International Order of the King's Daughters and Sons, by Sara R. Gugle.

Houses of Old Richmond, by Mary Wingfield Scott.

Medicine in Richmond, 1900-1975, by Charles M. Caravati, M.D.

Richmond After the War, 1865-1890, by Michael B. Chesson.

The Flair and the Fire: Story of the Episcopal Church in West Virginia, 1877-1977, by Eleanor Meyer Hamilton.

The Free Women of Petersburg: Status and Culture in a Southern Town, 1784-1860, by Suzanne Lebsock.

The History of Sheltering Arms Hospital, 1964, by Eda Carter Williams and Nita Ligon Morse.

The Social Transformation of American Medicine, by Paul Starr.

APPENDIX
Organizations and Administration

ADMINISTRATION

Richard C. Craven, *Executive Vice President and Administrator*
Henry H. Stonnington, M.D., *Vice President, Medical Affairs and Medical Director*
Michael J. McDonnell, *Vice President, Outpatient Services and Associate Administrator*
Richard W. Beckler, *Vice President, Financial Affairs*

PHYSICIANS REHABILITATION CLINIC

Albert M. Jones, M.D., *Associate Medical Director*
Manmohan S. Khokhar, M.D.
Jane Pendleton Wootton, M.D.

DEPARTMENT DIRECTORS
Centennial Year of 1989

Theresa Armstrong, *Therapeutic Recreation*
Gwen Avery, *Quality Assurance*
Nancy Barret, *Community/Volunteer Services*
Brenda Bartlett, *Environmental Services*
Anne Bullen, *Former Acting Director of Physical Therapy*
Sandy Gaskins, *Medical Records*
DiAnne Hambric, *Former Director of Personnel*
Marjorie Harrison, *Former Director of Nursing*
Wayne Humphries, *Public Relations*
Erma Kelley, *Speech Pathology/Audiology*
Karen Kelly, *Personnel*
Becky Mahler, *Social Work Services*
Michael Martelli, *Medical Psychology*
Irma Meade, *Nursing*
Robin Metcalf, *Former Director of Vocational Industrial Services*
Beverly Murphey, *Former Director of Therapeutic Recreation*
Sharon Nuzik, *Physical Therapy*
Doreen Schlimmer, *Vocational Industrial Services*
Judie Smith, *Occupational Therapy*
Valerie Young, *Day Rehabilitation Program*

BOARD OF DIRECTORS
Centennial Year of 1989

Rudolph H. Bunzl
Randolph B. Cardozo
Steven D. Delaney
Jean N. Dickinson, *president*
Virginia B. Hailes
Edwin L. Kendig, Jr., M.D.
Harry G. Lee, *vice president*
Anne R. Lower, *secretary*
Dale T. Mercer
J. Robert Nolley, Jr.
Stanley F. Pauley
C. Cotesworth Pinckney
John C. Purnell, Jr.
Heath K. Rada, Ed.D., *vice president*
William T. Reed III
John A. Robertson
Gilbert M. Rosenthal
S. Buford Scott
Nancy P. Thalhimer
Richard G. Tilghman
John D. Whitehurst, *treasurer*

ex officio:
Sally E. Flinn, *Women's Council president*

WOMEN'S COUNCIL

Centennial Year of 1989

Mrs. Edward C. Anderson
Mrs. Charles W. Appich, Jr., *treasurer*
Mrs. Wilson M. Brown, Jr.
Mrs. John H. Cecil, Jr., *second vice president*
Mrs. Todd Dabney
Mrs. Malcolm R. Dixon, Jr., *first vice president*
Mrs. William H. Emory, Jr.
Mrs. James B. Farinholt, Jr.
Mrs. Herbert E. Fitzgerald, Jr.
Mrs. James Flamming
Mrs. Lewis B. Flinn, Jr., *president*
Mrs. George H. Flowers, Jr.
Mrs. Kingsberry W. Gay, Jr., *Florence Nightingale Circle*
Mrs. Robert L. Gordon, Jr.
Mrs. William M. Hill
Mrs. Joseph A. Jennings
Mrs. James A. Jones, *assistant corresponding secretary*
Mrs. John F. Kay, Jr.
Mrs. Robert J. Keller III
Mrs. Lou S. Kendrick
Mrs. James E. Kulp, *Florence Nightingale Circle*
Mrs. Richard R. Lower
Mrs. J. Robert Massie, Jr.
Mrs. John L. McElroy
Mrs. Richard A. Michaux
Mrs. Edward F. Neal, Jr.
Mrs. William T. Nolley, *corresponding secretary*
Mrs. James F. Oates III
Mrs. Paul D. Sanders
Mrs. W. Holt Souder
Mrs. Thomas D. Stokes III, *Junior Board*
Mrs. Charles M. Terry, Jr.
Mrs. Morton G. Thalhimer, Jr.
Mrs. Julien H. Williams
Mrs. Mason M. Williams, *Junior Board*

GENERAL BOARD
Centennial Year of 1989

Mrs. Nancy Barret
FitzGerald Bemiss
Frederic S. Bocock
Arthur S. Brinkley, Jr.
Mrs. Henry A. Bullock, Jr.
Dr. Charles M. Caravati
Mrs. B. Noland Carter II
Robert Carter
Mrs. C. C. Chewning, Jr.
Mrs. Mary E. Chiles
Dixon W. Christian
Mrs. Herbert A. Claiborne, Jr.
James E. Covington, Jr.
Robert W. Daniel
Mrs. Ernest Edinger
Mrs. Maynard R. Emlaw
William H. Emory, Jr.
S. Douglas Fleet
Mrs. Robin A. Frayser
Mrs. Hiram T. Gates
Mrs. George D. Gibson
Mrs. Randolph W. Gunn, Jr.
Mrs. J. Pinckney Harrison
Mrs. DeWitt F. Helm, Jr.
Mrs. Walter Heubi
William M. Hill
Alfred R. Hunter
Mrs. Alfred R. Hunter
Kenneth R. Iseman
N. David Kjellstrom
Dr. Benjamin J. Lambert III
J. Clifford Miller, Jr.
Mrs. J. Clifford Miller, Jr.
Mrs. James Norwood
Mrs. W. Marshall Parrish III
John W. Pearsall, Sr.
Mrs. William R. Powell
Gordon F. Rainey, Jr.
Mrs. Edward Ray
William G. Reynolds, Jr.
Mrs. Franklin D. Robins
Mrs. John Robinson
Mrs. Calvin Satterfield
Mrs. James A. Saunders, Sr.
Walter W. Scott
Mrs. Helen P. Sterling
Everett W. Terrell
Mrs. Morton G. Thalhimer, Sr.
Morton G. Thalhimer, Jr.
E. Massie Valentine
Mrs. Luisa Whiting
Mrs. Walter A. Williams, Jr.

Epsilon Sigma Alpha Chapters
  Alpha Delta
  Alpha Tau
  Beta Beta
Florence Nightingale Circle
Friendship Club
Ginter Park Garden Club
Ginter Park Woman's Club
J.O.Y. Club of County Line Baptist Church
King's Daughters and Sons
  Fellowship Circle
  Wilma C. Cropper Circle
  Sheltering Arms Circle
Knights of Pythias
Ladies Sodality, St. Paul's Catholic Church
LaSertoma Club of Richmond
Newcomers Club of Richmond
PBX/Telecommunicators Club of Richmond
Richmond Rotary Club
Riverside Garden Club
Sertoma Club of Richmond
Stuart Avenue Community Relations Team (C & P)
Three Thousand Day Safety Club (DuPont)
TWERL Club

JUNIOR BOARD
Centennial Year of 1989

Mrs. John Mason Lee Antrim
Mrs. John F. Bain, Jr.
Mrs. Richard Kent Bennett
Mrs. Carl Fleming Blackwell
Mrs. Lawrence E. Blanchard III
Mrs. Andrew Mason Brent
Mrs. Thomas Rutherfoord Brown
Mrs. Trigg Brown
Mrs. Thomas Pinckney Bryan III
Mrs. John Kirkland Burke, Jr.
Mrs. B. Noland Carter III
Mrs. John Terry Cox
Mrs. John Hill Cronley III
Mrs. Francis Michael Crowley
Mrs. H. Aubrey Ford III
Mrs. John Paul Funkhouser
Mrs. John David Gottwald
Mrs. Baldwin Airey Hickey
Mrs. Wallace Brady Jones
Mrs. F. Claiborne Johnston, Jr.
Miss Elizabeth Law Keller
Mrs. Benjamin Rice Lacy IV, *vice president*
Mrs. William Evans Massey, Jr.
Mrs. George Riley Mercer, Jr.
Mrs. Claiborne Watkins Minor
Mrs. John Sanford Molster
Mrs. Douglas Durrell Monroe III
Mrs. Glenn Russell Moore
Mrs. Richard Wallace Nuckols, *Bal co-chairman*
Mrs. James Russell Parker III
Mrs. Robert Henry Pratt, *corresponding secretary*
Mrs. Theodore Winston Price
Mrs. Thomas T. Rankin
Mrs. Conrad F. Sauer IV
Mrs. George Ross Scott, *recording secretary*
Mrs. David G. Shuford
Mrs. Thomas D. Stokes III, *Bal co-chairman*
Mrs. Addison Baker Thompson
Mrs. Edward Hunter Thompson, Jr.
Mrs. Eugene Massie Valentine, Jr.
Mrs. Thomas Boushall Valentine
Mrs. Mason Miller Williams, *president*
Mrs. David Henry Worrell, Jr.
Mrs. Coleman Wortham II

BOARD OF DIRECTORS PRESIDENTS

1892-1904	C. V. Meredith
1904-1911	D. O. Davis
1912-1925	E. B. Addison
1925-1932	A. D. Williams
1932-1939	Frederic W. Scott
1939-1940	Legh R. Page
1940-1945	Buford Scott
1945-1947	W. Frank Powers
1947-1952	James H. Scott
1952-1955	William T. Reed, Jr.
1955-1957	Morton G. Thalhimer
1957-1960	John S. Davenport III
1960-1962	Robert Carter
1962-1965	Arthur S. Brinkley, Jr.
1965-1967	Morton G. Thalhimer, Jr.
1967-1969	Robert L. Gordon, Jr.
1969-1972	S. Buford Scott
1972-1974	William T. Reed III
1974-1976	Randolph B. Cardozo
1976-1978	Randolph W. McElroy
1978-1980	Arthur M. Hungerford, Jr.
1980-1983	Gordon F. Rainey, Jr.
1983-1985	Anne R. Lower (Mrs. Richard R.)
1985-1986	Dixon W. Christian
1986-1988	C. Cotesworth Pinckney
1988-1990	Jean N. Dickinson (Mrs. Enders III)

EXECUTIVE BOARD PRESIDENTS

1892-1895	Mrs. J. H. Claiborne
1896-1897	Miss Jane Rutherford
	Mrs. E. B. Addison
1897-1899	Mrs. Frances Deane Williams
1900-1910	Mrs. Joshua Peterkin
1911-1937	Miss Frances Branch Scott
1937-1938	Mrs. George T. King
1938-1945	Mrs. Ramon Garcin
1945-1947	Mrs. W. Brooke Catlett
1948-1950	Mrs. Edward Clifford Anderson
1951-1953	Mrs. William Frazier

BOARD OF MANAGERS PRESIDENTS

1953-1955 Mrs. Walter A. Williams, Jr.
1955-1958 Mrs. John Lee McElroy
1958-1960 Mrs. Richard A. Michaux
1960-1962 Mrs. Thomas F. Wheeldon
1962 Mrs. John H. Cecil, Jr.
1962-1963 Mrs. Thomas Nelson Williams
1963-1964 Mrs. Richard A. Michaux
1964-1966 Mrs. George H. Flowers, Jr.
1966-1968 Mrs. William H. Emory, Jr.
1968-1970 Mrs. W. Holt Souder
1970-1972 Mrs. Randolph W. Gunn, Jr.
1972-1974 Mrs. Robert J. Keller III
1974-1976 Mrs. George H. Flowers, Jr.
1976-1978 Mrs. Charles M. Terry, Jr.
1978-1979 Mrs. Todd Dabney
1979-1980 Mrs. DeWitt F. Helm, Jr.

WOMEN'S COUNCIL PRESIDENTS

1980-1981 Mrs. DeWitt F. Helm, Jr.
1981-1982 Mrs. John F. Kay, Jr.
1982-1984 Mrs. Morton G. Thalhimer, Jr.
1984-1986 Mrs. Charles W. Appich, Jr.
1986-1988 Mrs. Todd Dabney
1988-1990 Mrs. Lewis B. Flinn, Jr.

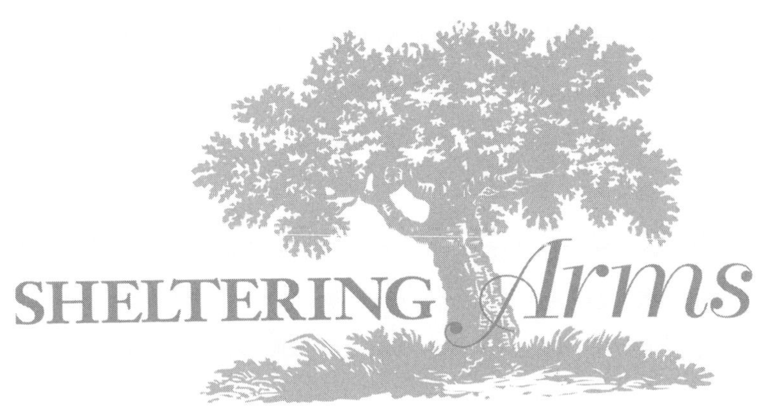

the Next Fifteen Years

THE MISSION of Sheltering Arms Physical Rehabilitation Hospital is to provide comprehensive physical rehabilitation of the highest caliber with compassion and respect, to enhance the quality of life for those persons experiencing disabilities, and to offer financial assistance to those in need.

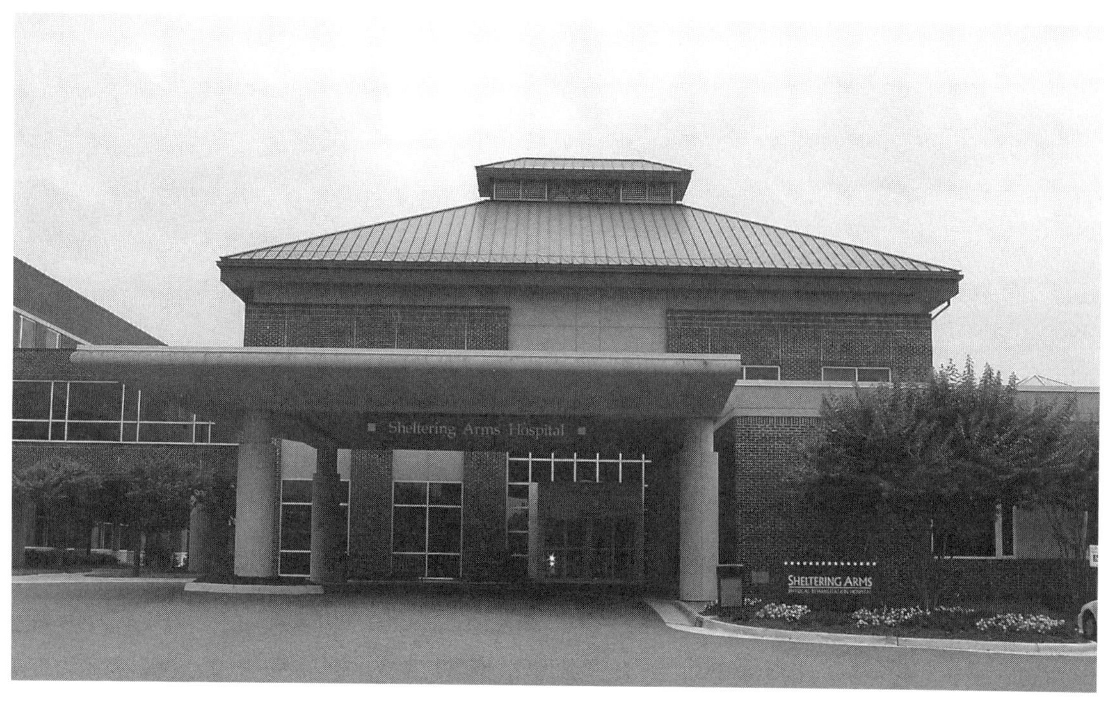

Sheltering Arms has been able to change as needs in the community have changed. In 1998, the Hospital moved to the campus of the Bon Secours Memorial Regional Medical Center in Mechanicsville under the direction of CEO Richard Craven. With 40 private rooms, it is physically connected to the acute care hospital. A full range of rehabilitation services is offered to inpatients. Outpatient neurorehab and orthopaedic/spine therapies are also offered on the campus.

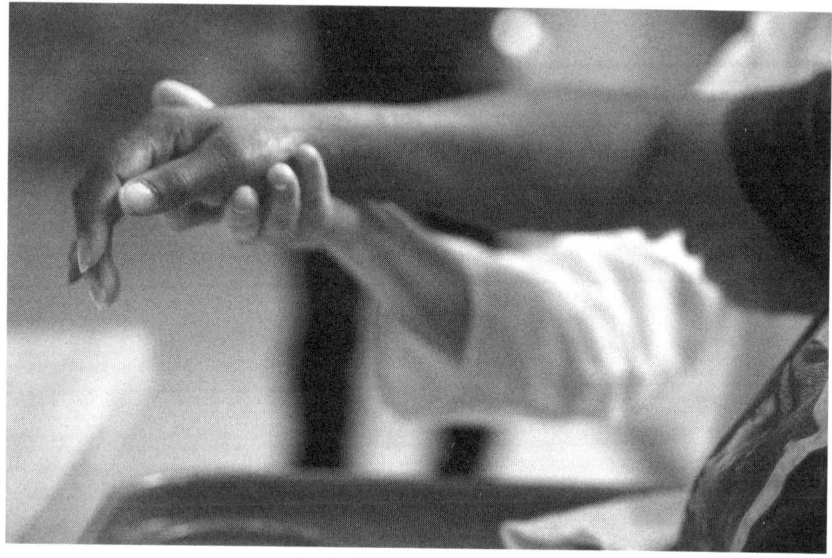

RICHARD USTINICH

If this desk is unattended,
please go to the window
on your right for assistance

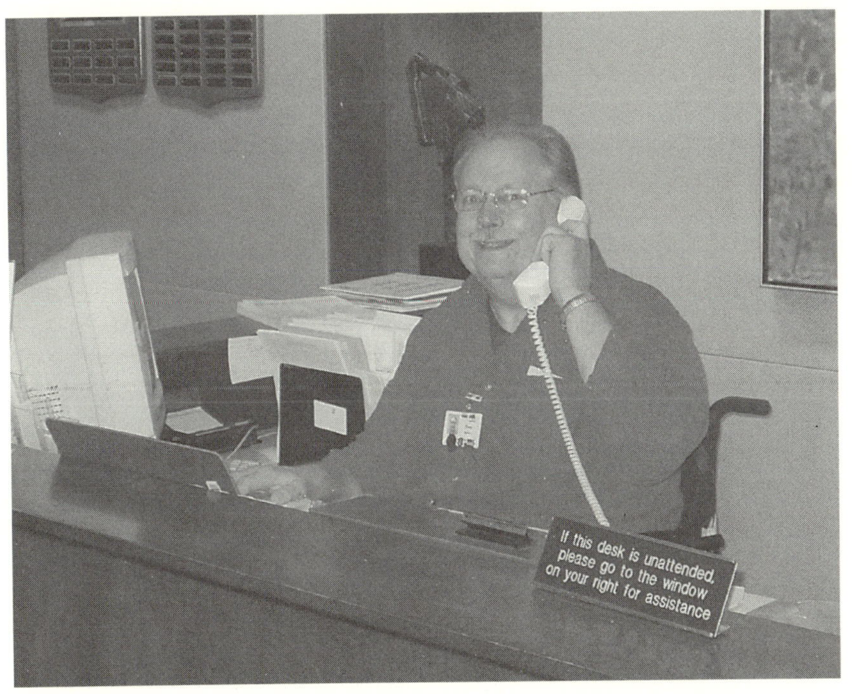

Volunteers continue to play an important role at Sheltering Arms. Tom Horne has been greeting patients and visitors at the front desk since 1989.

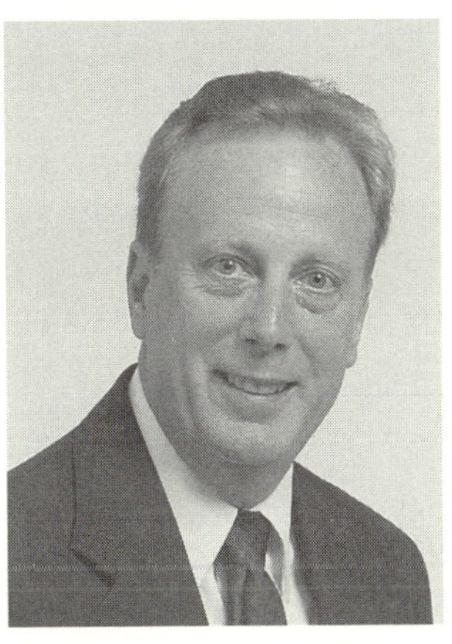

Dr. Jack Carroll became CEO and President in September 1998 and leads a staff of over 500 professionals in Sheltering Arms locations throughout Central Virginia.

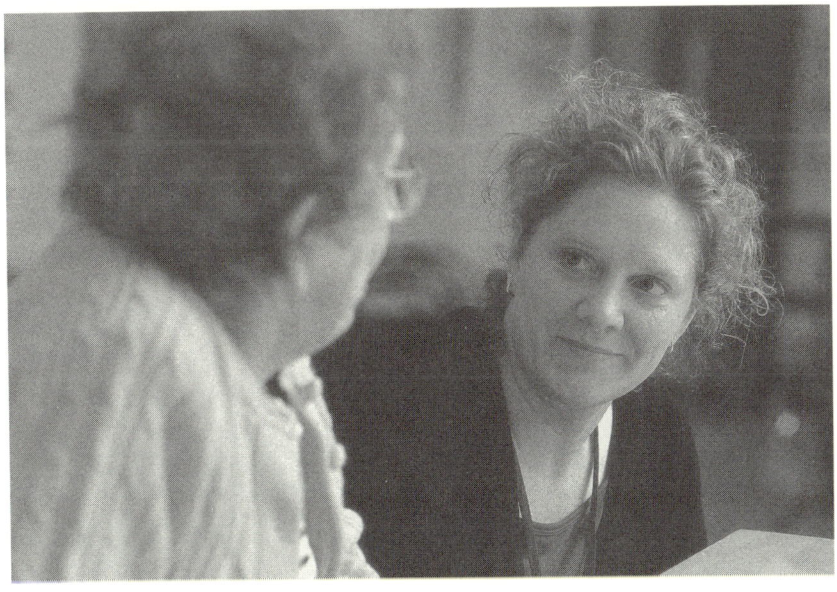

RICHARD USTINICH

Staff at Sheltering Arms are committed to showing patients the difference that caring can make.

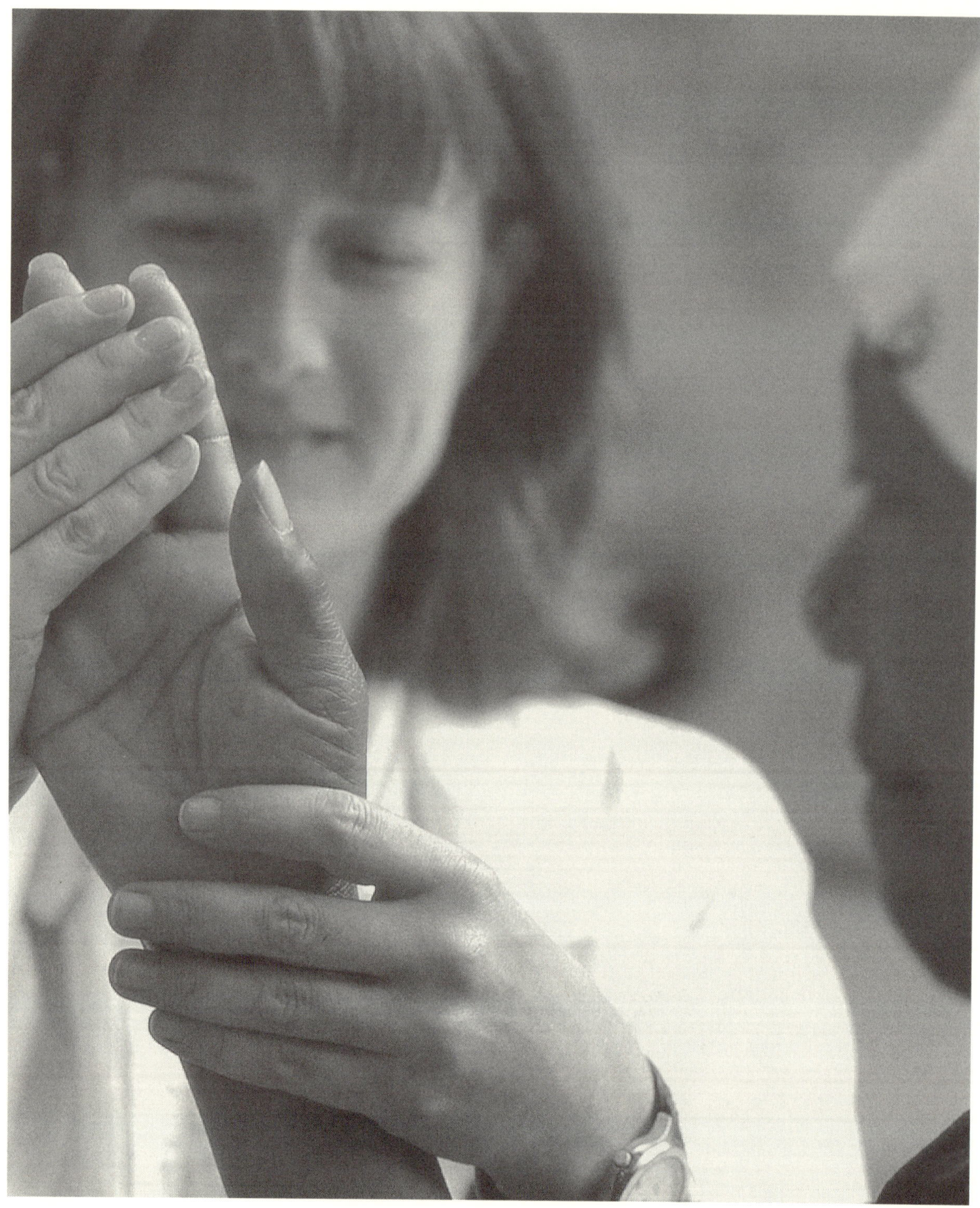

RICHARD USTINICH

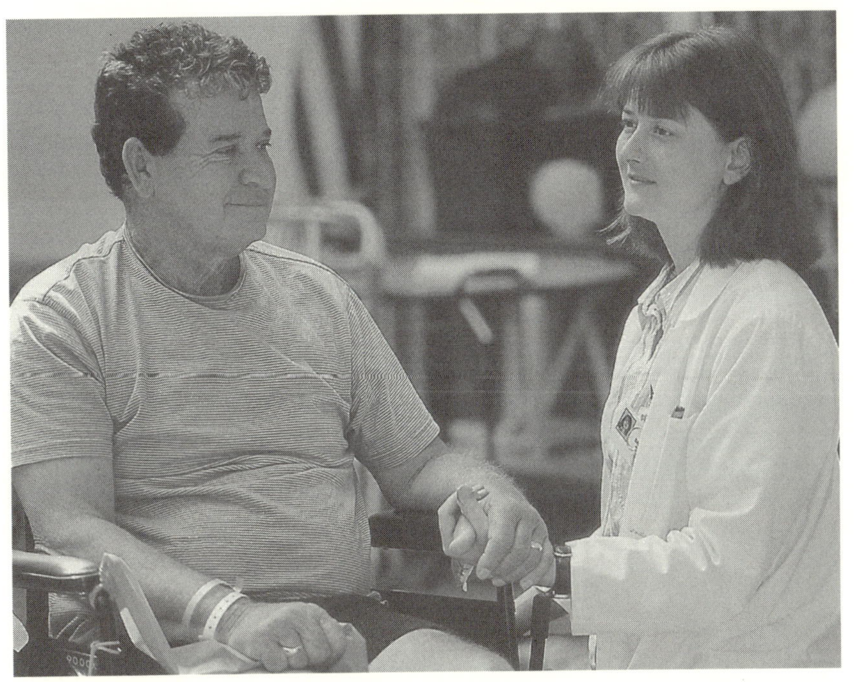

RICHARD USTINICH

Every patient comes to Sheltering Arms with a different story. And yet, they all share a common driving desire: to re-engage with life. At Sheltering Arms, we help make this happen.

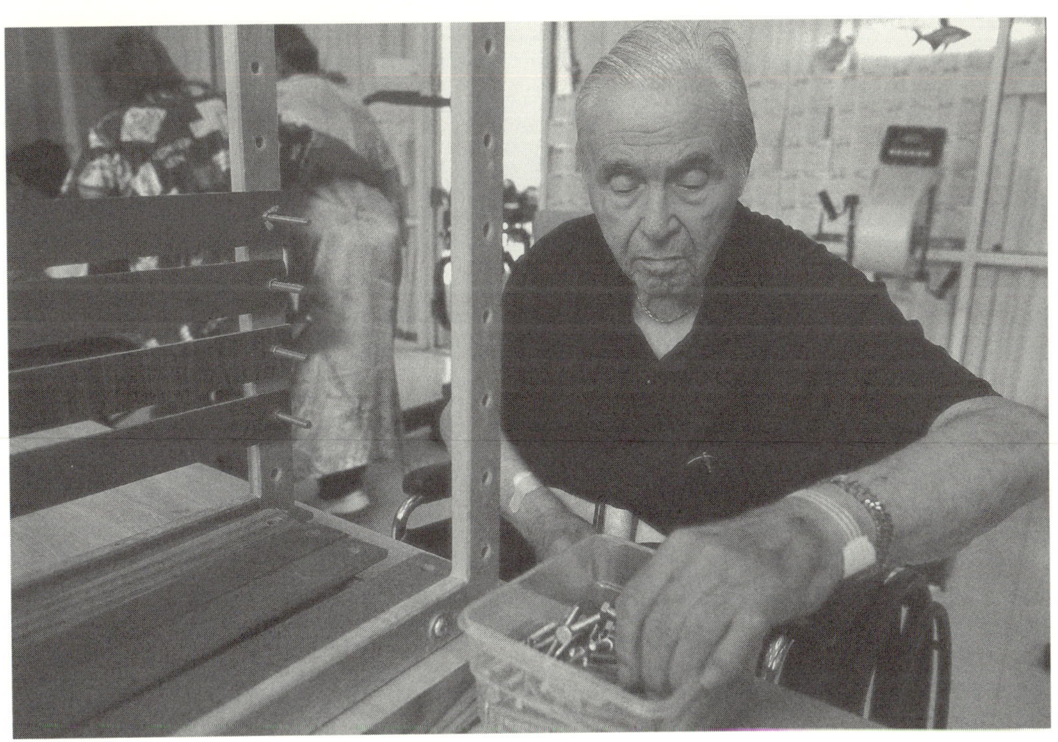

RICHARD USTINICH

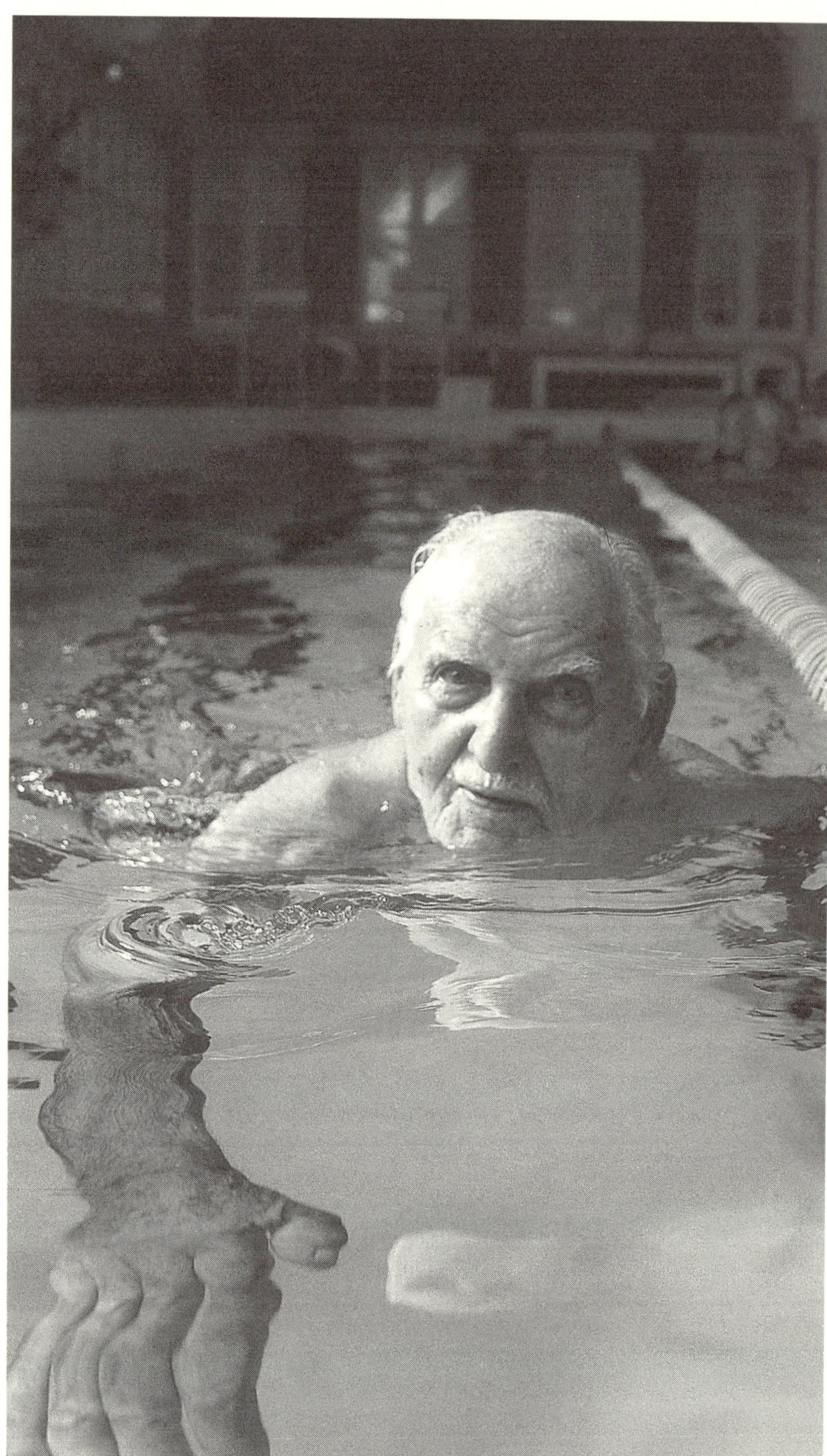

RICHARD USTINICH

Sheltering Arms is dedicated to empowering people to embrace a lifetime of recreation and wellness. Through wellness classes, special events, our unique Club Rec program and pool and fitness memberships, Sheltering Arms' commitment to the patients does not end when therapy services are completed.

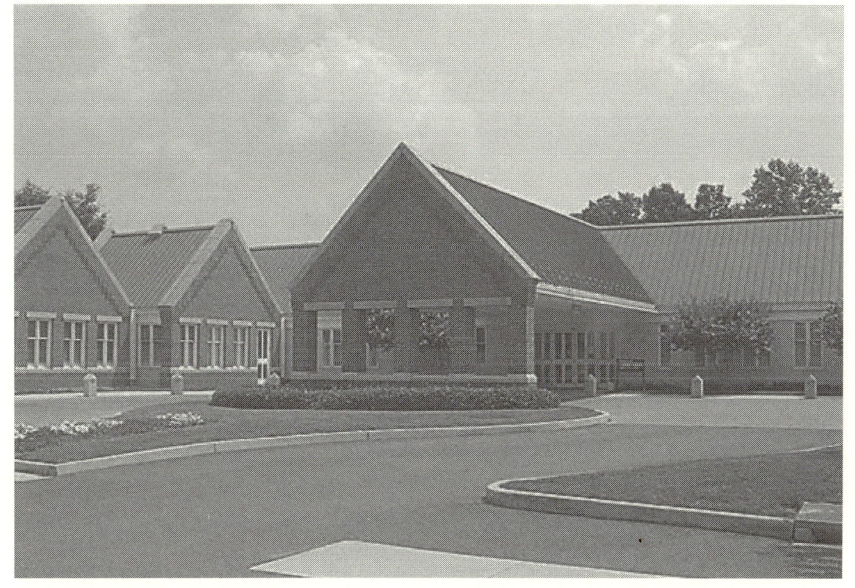

The Day Rehab Program, previously located in Stony Point, is now located at the Sheltering Arms Bon Air location at 206 Twinridge Lane. This is also the location of the business office, warm water therapeutic pool and a wheelchair accessible fitness center.

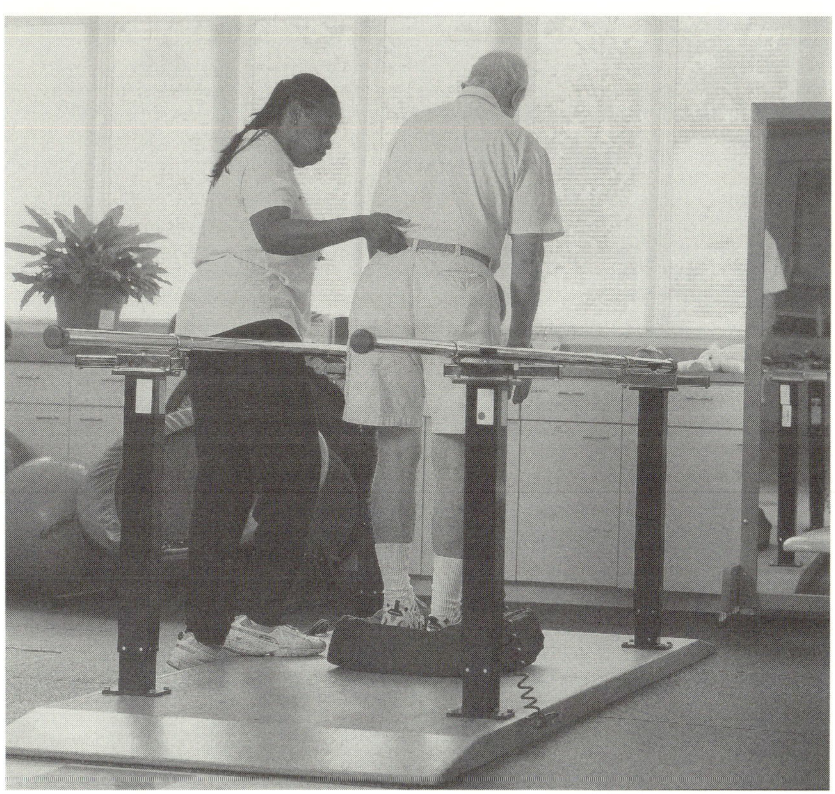

Sheltering Arms outpatient services are offered at clinics throughout the greater Richmond area to meet the needs of the growing community.

RICHARD USTINICH

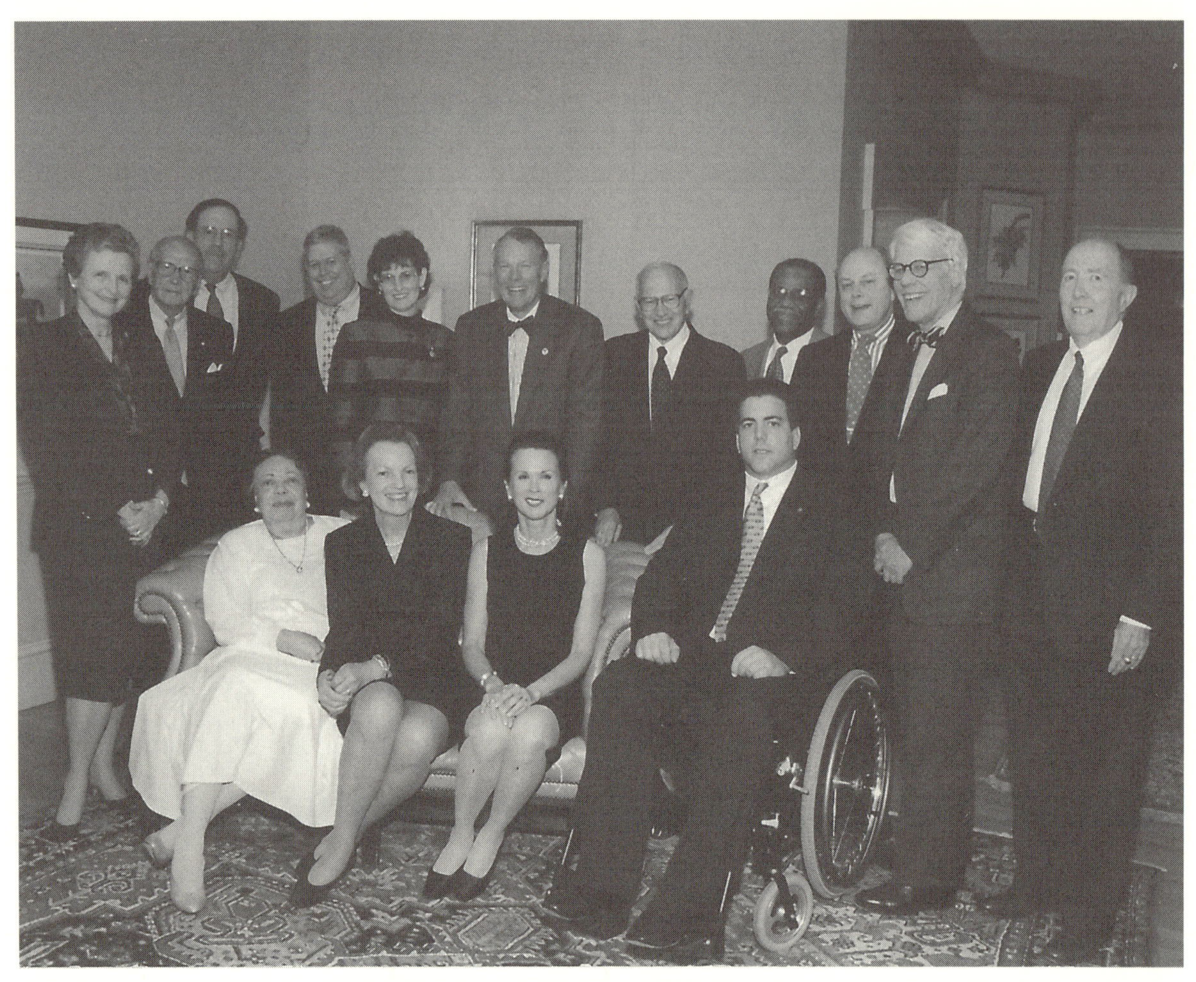

1998 Board of Directors

Seated:
Verdelle Bradley, Annabel Josephs, President, *Dale Mercer, Gary Melton*

Standing:
Anne Lower, Dr. E.L. Kendig, Bates Chappell, Dr. Heath Rada, Patricia Cushnie, Buford Scott, Gilbert Rosenthal, John Purnell, Dr. Donald Switz, Cotesworth Pinckney, John Robertson

Not Present:
Arthur Brinkley, Thomas Cunningham, Steven Delaney, Dr. Peter Goodman, Dr. Laurie Rennie, Carter Scott

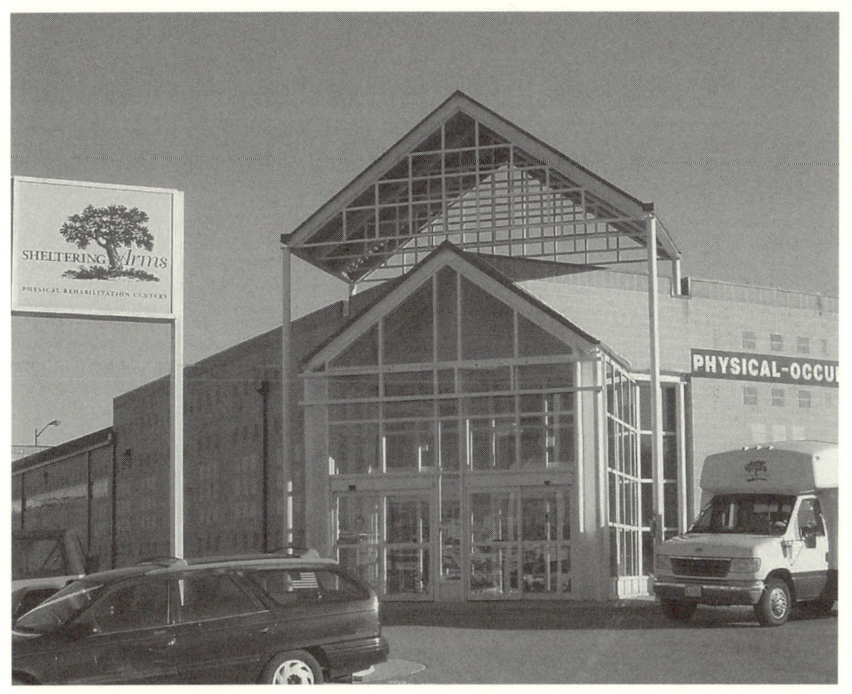

To complete the continuum of rehabilitative services, Sheltering Arms offers the Club Rec program at the Midtown location near the intersection of Broad Street and the Boulevard.

An active program for exercise, spiritual enrichment, service to the community and adaptive recreational events, such as the annual golf tournament, Club Rec is focused on embracing life following illness or injury. Members even take overnight cruises!

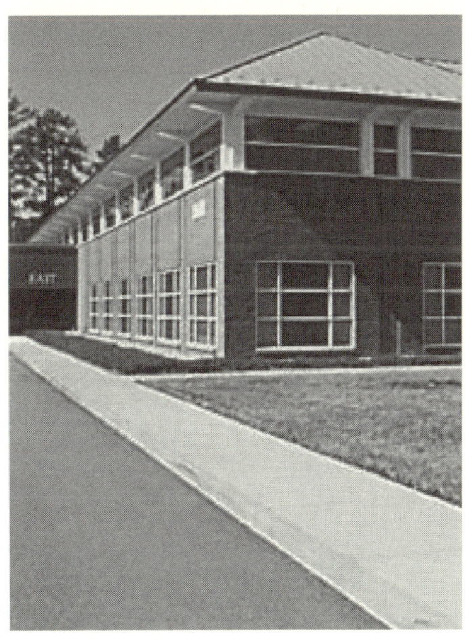

Reaching out to the Richmond suburbs, another outpatient clinic is located at 11601 Ironbridge Road in Chester.

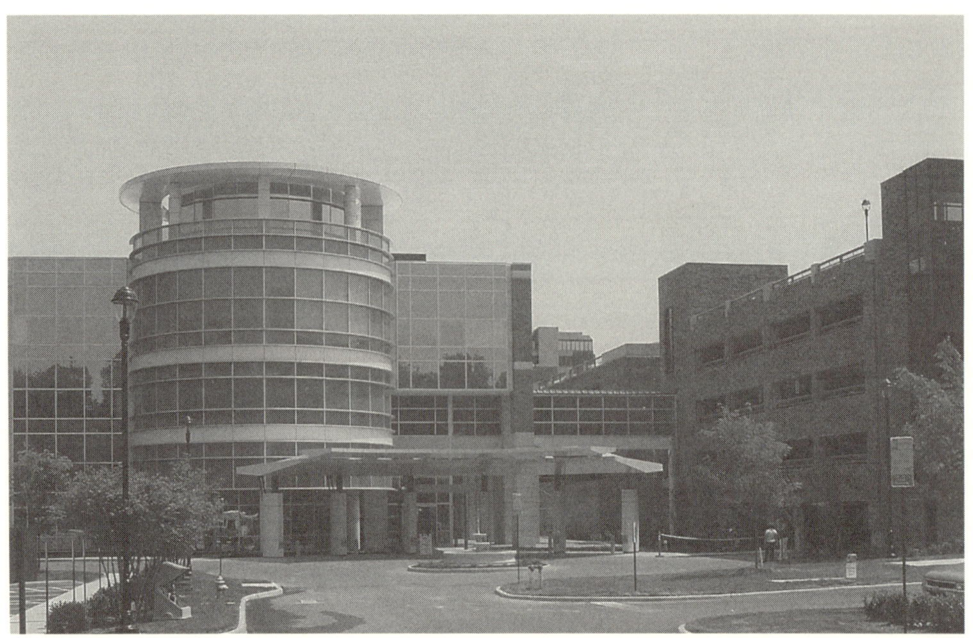

The Sheltering Arms Spine and Sport Center is located on the growing St. Mary's Hospital campus in Henrico County. Clinicians at this site specialize in helping patients with orthopaedic conditions. The Spine and Sport Center also offers a fitness center and a sports performance enhancement program, called Acceleration Richmond.

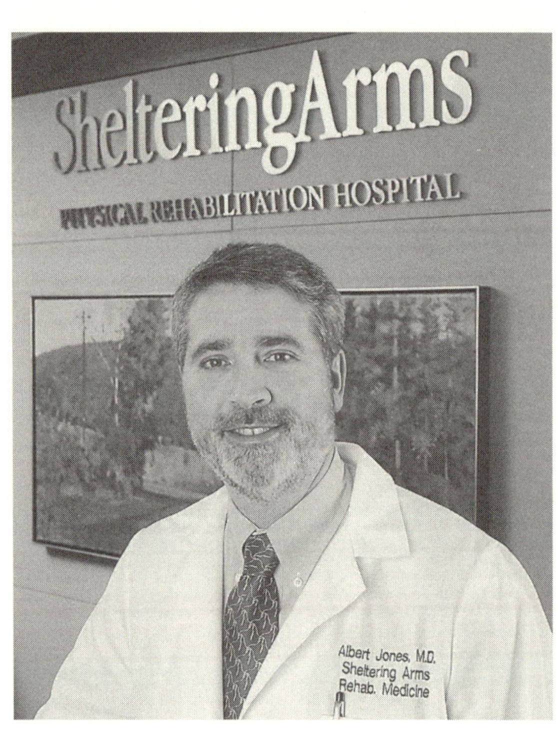

ALLEN JONES

Dr. Albert M. Jones, Jr. joined Sheltering Arms in 1988 and serves as Medical Director.

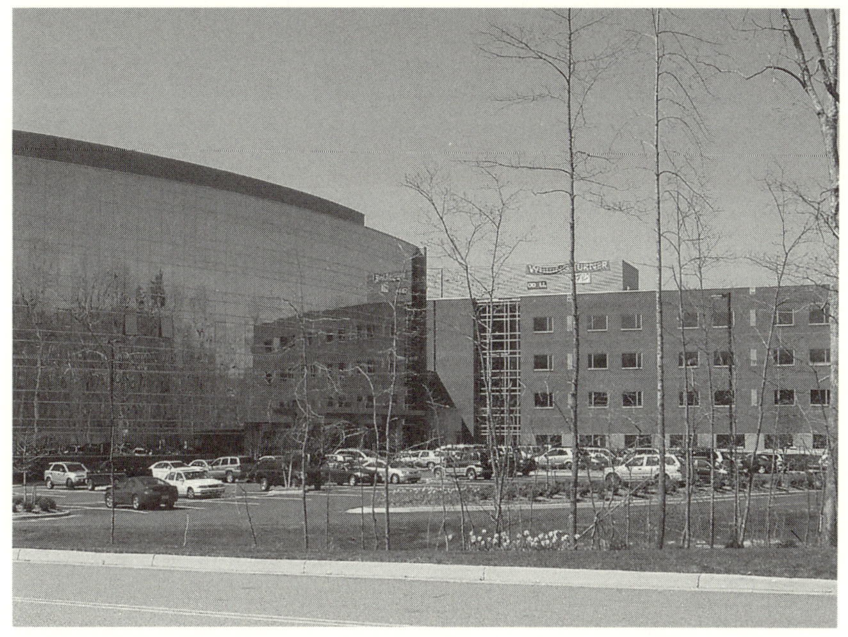

Again to meet the needs of this growing area, Sheltering Arms Hospital South opened in November 2005 offering 28 inpatient rehabilitation beds on the campus of St. Francis Medical Center in Midlothian. The hospital is located on the fourth floor of the Medical Office Building.

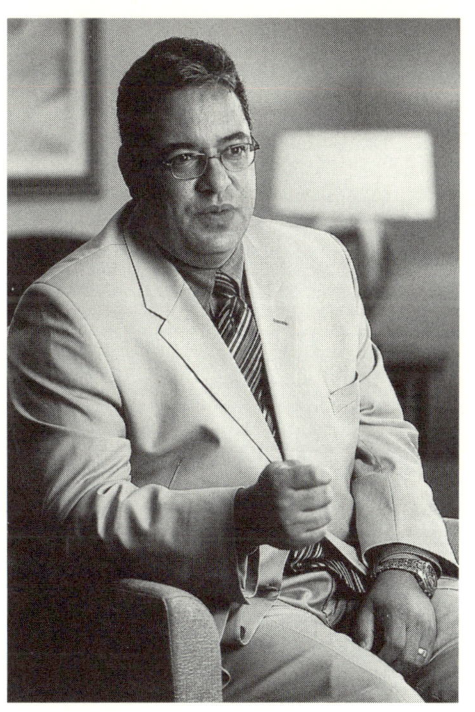

RICHARD USTINICH

Dr. Timothy Silver serves as the Medical Director for Sheltering Arms Hospital South.

Outpatient therapy and physician services are also offered on the St. Francis campus on the third floor of the Medical Office Building.

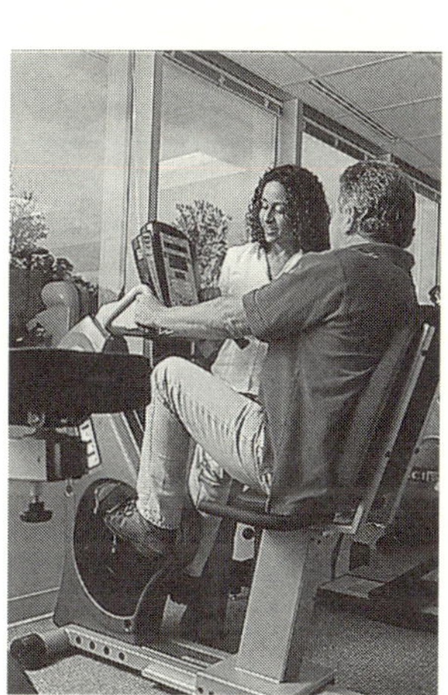

RICHARD USTINICH

Sheltering Arms Staff 2006

SENIOR ADMINISTRATION

Jack Carroll, Ph.D., MHA, *President and Chief Executive Officer*
Michael McDonnell, *Vice President and Chief Operating Officer*
Richard Beckler, *Vice President and Chief Financial Officer, 1986-2006*
Greg Spruill, *Vice President and Chief Financial Officer, 2006-forward*
Albert Jones, Jr., M.D., *Medical Director*
Cheryl Lee-Roznowski, *Associate Vice President of Inpatient Services and Chief Nurse Executive*
James Braith, *Associate Vice President of Professional Services*
Kelly Lewis, *Associate Vice President of Human Resources*

PHYSICIANS

Albert Jones, Jr., M.D., *Medical Director*
Michael DePalma, M.D.
C. Matthew Gibellato, M.D.
Hillary Hawkins, M.D.
Michael Lane, M.D.
Gregory Leghart, M.D.
Timothy Silver, M.D., *Medical Director, Sheltering Arms Hospital South*
Yaoming Gu, M.D.
David X. Cifu, M.D., *Chairman, VCU Department of Physical Medicine and Rehabilitation*
Karen Steidle, M.D.

DIRECTORS

Alison Clarke, *Director of Community Recreation Services*
Jennifer Sheppard, *Director of Special Projects*
José Vivaldi, *Director of Outpatient Services*
Cindy High, *Director of the Business Office*
Naomi Waddy, *Director of Patient Accounting*
Pam Meadows, *Director of Nursing*
Richard Peay, *Director of Patient Access*
Rod Edwards, *Director of Materials Management*
Sandra Gaskins, *Director of Medical Records*
Shawne Soper, *Director of Contract Services*
Travis Gathright, *Director of Information Technology*

2006 BOARD OF DIRECTORS

Patricia B. Cushnie, R.N., *Chairman*
John Lee McElroy III, *First Vice President*
Joyce Nash, *Second Vice President*
W. Bates Chappell, *Treasurer*
Evans B. Brasfield, *Secretary*
Ronald Bargatze
Cathryn Barley
Andy Bennett
Vickie W. Blanchard
Charles M. Caravati III
William T. Clarke, Jr.
Lawrence E. Gibson
Melanie Goodpasture
William E. Hardy
John M. O'Bannon III, M.D.
C. Cotesworth Pinckney
Lisa Taylor Powell
Theodore W. Price
Corbin Kendig Rankin
Dianne Reynolds-Cane, M.D.
Donald M. Switz, M.D., *Immediate Past Chairman*
Holly Antrim, *Women's Council President*
Marietta Reynolds, *Junior Board President*

BOARD OF DIRECTORS CHAIRMEN

1990-1992	Harry G. Lee
1992-1994	Rudolph H. Bunzl
1994-1996	Steven D. Delaney
1996-1998	John A. Robertson
1998-2000	Annabel S. Josephs, R.N.
2000-2002	R. Carter Scott III
2002-2004	John C. Purnell, Jr.
2004-2006	Donald M. Switz, M.D.
2006	Patricia B. Cushnie, R.N.

WOMEN'S COUNCIL 2006

Holly Antrim, *President*
Nell Thompson, *Vice President*
Nancy Barret, *Corresponding Secretary*
Helga Boyan, *Treasurer*
Jean Appich
Andy Bennett
Vickie Blanchard
Lilliboo Cronly
Molly Fitzgerald
Sally Flinn
Anne Lower
Julia Gray Michaux
Caroline Morton
Johnnie Lou Terry
Pattie Williams
Vann Williams
Marietta Reynolds, *Junior Board President*
Kathy Jones, *Secretary*

WOMEN'S COUNCIL PRESIDENTS

1990-1992	Mrs. Malcolm R. Dixon, Jr.
1992-1994	Mrs. Wilson M. Brown, Jr.
1994-1996	Mrs. Mason N. Williams
1996-1998	Mrs. Horace Wright
1998-2000	Mrs. Lawrence Blanchard
2000-2003	Mrs. Richard K. Bennett
2003-2005	Mrs. Marshall N. Morton
2005	Mrs. John Mason Antrim

GENERAL BOARD

Mrs. Nancy S. Barret
FitzGerald Bemiss (Honorary)
Mrs. John D. Blair
Frederic C. Bocock
Mrs. Wilson M. Brown, Jr.
Mrs. B. Noland Carter II
Mrs. John H. Cecil
Mrs. C.C. Chewning, Jr.
Mrs. Mary E. Chiles
Dixon W. Christian
Mrs. Herbert A. Claiborne, Jr.
Mrs. Isabel Souder Correll
James E. Covington, Jr.
Mrs. Todd Dabney
Robert W. Daniel
Mrs. Virginia Brent Evans
Mrs. George H. Flowers, Jr.
Mrs. Robin S. Frayser
Mrs. George D. Gibson
Mrs. Mary Jones Helm
William M. Hill
Mrs. William M. Hill
Mrs. Alfred R. Hunter
Mrs. Carolyn Johnston
Mrs. John F. Kay, Jr.
Mrs. Robert J. Keller III
N. David Kjellstrom
Mrs. Benjamin R. Lacy III
Dr. Benjamin J. Lambert III
Mrs. J. Clifford Miller, Jr.
Mrs. Richard Morrill
Mrs. James F. Oates III
John W. Pearsall, Sr.
Gordon F. Rainey, Jr.
Mrs. Bettie Roach
Mrs. Calvin Satterfield III
Walter W. Scott
Mrs. Sidney L. Stern II
Mrs. Charles R. Stitzer, Jr.
Mrs. Thomas D. Stokes
Morton G. Thalhimer, Jr.
Mrs. Morton G. Thalhimer, Jr.
Richard G. Tilghman
E. Massie Valentine
Miss L. Elizabeth Walton
Mrs. Louisa Whiting
Mrs. Julien H. Williams
Ms. Brenda Wiltshire

Epsilon Sigma Alpha Sorority
  Alpha Delta Chapter
  Alpha Tau Chapter
Ginter Park Garden Club
Ginter Park Woman's Club
J.O.Y. Club of County Line
  Baptist Church
Junior Board of SA
King's Daughters and Sons
  Fellowship Circle
  Wilma C. Cropper Circle
  Sheltering Arms Circle
Knights of Pythias
Ladies Sodality of St. Paul's
  Catholic Church
Hands of Friendship Club
PBX/Telecommunications Club
  of Richmond
Richmond Rotary Club
Riverside Garden Club
Richmond on the James
  Sertoma Club
3000 Day Safety Club
  of DuPont
Women's Council of SA

JUNIOR BOARD 2006

Mrs. Wyatt S. Beazley IV
Mrs. J. Ros Bowers
Mrs. Peter K. Braden
Mrs. Turner Bredrup
Mrs. Austin Brockenbrough IV
Mrs. Lynnie Brugh
Mrs. Charles Caravati III
Mrs. Tazwell M. Carrington IV
Mrs. Dean Caven
Mrs. Herbert A. Claiborne III
Mrs. William W. Clarkson, Jr.
Mrs. Thorp J. Davis
Mrs. J. Clifford Foster IV
Mrs. W. Hill Griffin
Mrs. Lee P. Hatcher, *Bal Co-Chairman*
Mrs. Clay Hilbert
Mrs. John Gwyn Jordan III
Mrs. Dean King
Mrs. David Lyons
Mrs. William Richmond McDaniel
Mrs. Duncan Alexander MacLeod
Mrs. Thurston Moore
Mrs. Stewart O'Keefe
Mrs. John D. O'Neill, Jr.
Mrs. Julian Ottley
Mrs. Houghton Phillips
Mrs. Charles Plageman
Mrs. Charles M. Polk III
Mrs. Benjamin Watkins Rawles III, *Bal Co-Chairman*
Mrs. Alexander Reeves
Mrs. Bagley Reid
Mrs. Richard Samuel Reynolds, *President*
Mrs. Edward P. Roberts
Mrs. Christopher W. Rusbuldt
Mrs. Charles M. Stillwell, *First Vice President*
Mrs. John Ballard Syer
Mrs. William St. Clair Talley
Mrs. Edward West Valentine
Mrs. John Wallace
Mrs. Scott Wallace
Mrs. Peter Thornton Wilbanks
Mrs. Christopher H. Williams
Mrs. David Wise
Mrs. Murray H. Wright

COLOPHON

SHELTERING ARMS HOSPITAL: *A Centennial History (1898-1998), with Updates through 2006,* was set in Palatino and Michelangelo.

Original linocuts by Jack A. Molloy. Book design by Tina Brubaker Chovanec and Linda Berry / Designer's Ink.

Printed and bound by The American Book Company, Don J. Beville, Publisher.

Typographical revisions by I. Todd Stanley.